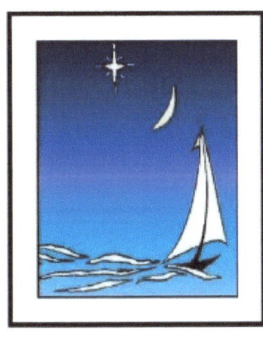

Sleep
ePortal

A Sleep Disorders Reference for Physicians
1st Edition, 2006

Liam Alexander Briones MD
Editors: Joseph Sopko MD
Kingman Strohl MD.

Author:
Liam Alexander Briones, MD, MBA, FCCP, FAASM
Senior Clinical Instructor, Case Western Reserve University
Medical Director Pulmonary Services, St. Vincent Charity Hospital
Medical Director Sleep Disorders Center, St. Vincent Charity Hospital,
    Cleveland, OH
Author and Developer, MDePortal electronic medical record and website.
Chief Editor, ICU ePortal
Member, American Academy Sleep Medicine, American Thoracic Society,
    Society of Critical Care Medicine
Alumni Executive MBA program, University of Tennessee, 2002

Editors:
Joseph Sopko, MD
Assistant Professor of Medicine, Department of Medicine,
    Case Western Reserve University.
Adjunct Faculty, Cuyahoga Community College
Director, Department of Medicine, St. Vincent Charity Hospital
Director, Medical Intensive Care Unit, St. Vincent Charity Hospital,
    January 1981 to present
Respiratory Therapy Advisory Committee, Cuyahoga Community College,
    1980 to present
Board of Medical Consultants, Cleveland Police, 1987 to present
Member, Executive Committee, American Lung Association of Northern Ohio,
    1995 to present
Member, Medical Moral Advisory Group, Diocese of Cleveland, 1994 to present
Member, Clinical Quality Improvement Committee, Medical Mutual of Ohio,
    1997 to present
Member, Risk Management Committee, Medical Mutual of Ohio, 1997 to present
Consultant, Pneumonia Project, Ke-PRO, 1999 to present

Kingman Strohl, MD
Director, Centers for Sleep Disorders Research
Professor of Medicine, Case Western Reserve University
Professor of Anatomy, Case Western Reserve University

*ICD-9 codes from the International Classification of Sleep Disorders in parenthesis.

Disclaimer: The field of sleep is rapidly evolving and there may be many updates published at the time of the Sleep ePortal release that are not included in this edition. This manuscript is intended to provide a base to guide you in the diagnosis and management of sleep problems encountered in clinical practice. It is intended to be a point of care tool in the day to day activities related to sleep, from assessing and managing patients, to billing and coding and to understanding or interpreting sleep studies. You may keep it on your desk top or on your hand held device to assist you at the bedside. You may review the table of contents to identify subjects of interest or use the search or find feature from the File menu of Acrobat Reader to find key words.   I hope you find it helpful. I welcome feedback. You may write at drliam16@gmail.com. Thank you.

Warmest Regards,

Liam Alexander Briones MD, MBA, FAASM, FCCP, FCP, FSCCM, PScD, ABAARM, FAAARM.
November 30, 2016

*ICD-9 codes from the International Classification of Sleep Disorders in parenthesis.

PROLOGUE:

I am so proud to be a member of St. Vincent Charity
Hospital, an organization that houses Cuyahoga
County's only 24-hour Psychiatric Emergency
Department, and I dedicate this book to the everyday
heroes who bravely struggle with mental illness, their families and
the professionals who spend each day improving the
lives of those who suffer.

With proper treatment, people living with mental
illnesses can lead full and productive lives. However,
recent cuts in mental health care funding have led to
a crisis situation. Those who would benefit most from
community services are falling through the cracks
without treatment or proper resources. Those of us who have been
blessed with physical and mental health have the opportunity to share
our gifts with those who through no fault of their own experience the
trauma of mental illness. This book's profits are dedicated to raise
funds for the St. Vincent Charity Hospital Psychiatric Emergency
Department. Additional contributions
to the Psychiatric Emergency Department at SVCH are
greatly encouraged. With your generous support, the
Psychiatric Emergency Department can continue to
provide services so that those struggling can control
their mental illness and reach their personal goals.

Warmest regards,

Liam Alexander Briones MD, MBA, FCCP, FAASM.

*ICD-9 codes from the International Classification of Sleep Disorders in parenthesis.

SLEEP ePORTAL CONTENT:

SLEEP DISORDERS CLASSIFICATION
I. *PARASOMNIAS*
1. NON-REM PARASOMNIAS
1.1 Disorders of Arousals: Confusional arousals (307.46-2), Sleep Walking (307.46-0), sleep terrors (307.46.1), Sleep-related eating (780.52-8).
2. PRIMARY MISCELLANEOUS SLEEP PHENOMENA
Bruxism (306.8), Enuresis (780.56-0), rhythmic movement Disorder (307.3), Periodic Leg Movement Disorder (PLM) (780.52.4), Sleep Talking (307.47-3).
3. REM PARASOMNIAS
3.1 Sinus Arrest (780.56-8)
3.2 REM behavior disorder (RBD) (780.59-0)
3.3 Nightmares(307.47-0)
3.4 Sleep Paralysis (780.56-2)
3.5 Impaired sleep-related penile erections (780.56-3)
3.6 Sleep related painful erections (780.56-4)
4. SLEEP-WAKE TRANSITION DISORDERS
4.1 Rhythmic Movement Disorder (307.3)
4.2 Sleep Starts (307.47-2)
4.3 Sleep Talking (307.47-3)
4.4 Nocturnal Leg Cramps (729.82)

II. *DYSSOMNIAS*
II.1.1 Psycho physiologic insomnia (307.42-0)
II.1.2 Sleep State misperception (307.49-1)
II.1.3 Idiopathic insomnia (780.52-7)
II.1.4 Narcolepsy (347)
II.1.5 Idiopathic hypersomnia(780.54-7)
II.1.6 Recurrent hypersomnia (780.54-2)
II.1.7 Posttraumatic hypersomnia (780.54-8) 6
II.1.8 Obstructive Sleep Apnea (OSA) (780.53-0)
II.1.9 Central Sleep Apnea Syndrome   (CSA) (780.51-1)
II.1.10 Central Alveolar Hypoventilation (CAH) (780.51-1)
II.1.11 Periodic Limb Movement Disorder (PLMD) (780.52-4)
II.1.12 Restless Legs Syndrome (RLS) (780.52-5)
II.2 Intrinsic sleep Disorder NOS
II.3 Extrinsic sleep Disorders: Inadequate sleep hygiene (307.41-1), Environmental sleep disorder (780.52-6), Altitude insomnia (289.0), Adjustment sleep disorder (307.41-0), Insufficient sleep syndrome (307.49-4), limit-setting sleep disorder (307.42-4), Sleep-onset association disorder (307.42-5), Food allergy insomnia (780.52-2), Nocturnal eating (drinking) syndrome (780.52-8), hypnoptic-dependent sleep disorder

*ICD-9 codes from the International Classification of Sleep Disorders in parenthesis.

(780.52-8), stimulant-dependent sleep disorder (780.52-1), alcohol-dependent sleep disorder (780.52-3), Toxin-induced sleep disorder (780.54-6), extrinsic sleep disorder NOS.

II.4 Circadian Rhythm Sleep Disorders: Time zone change (jet lag) syndrome (307.45-0), shift work sleep disorder (307.45-1), Irregular sleep-wake pattern (307.45-3), Delayed sleep phase syndrome (780.55-0), Advanced sleep phase syndrome (780.55-1), Non-24 hour sleep-wake disorder (780.55-2)

III. SECONDARY SLEEP PHENOMENA
1. Neurological
1.1 Primary Headache
1.2 Secondary Headache
1.3 Fatal Familial Insomnia (337.9)
1.4 Sleep Related Epilepsy (345), Electrical Status Epilepticus of Sleep (345.8)
1.5 Cerebral degenerative Disorders
1.6 Dementia (331)
1.7 Parkinsonism (332-333)
2. Cardio-Pulmonary Sleep Phenomena: Sinus arrest, Angina (411-414), Asthma/COPD (490-494), sleep related asthma (493), abnormal swallowing, sleep –related laryingospasm, primary snoring.
3. Gastrointestinal: Gastroesophageal Reflux (GERD) (530.1), Diffuse esophageal spasm
4. Miscellaneous
4.1 Nocturnal Muscle Cramps
4.2 Nocturnal Paroxysmal Dystonia (PND)(780.59-)
4.3 Sudden unexplained death syndrome (SUDS) (780.59-3)
4.4 Benign neonatal sleep myoclonus(780.59-5)
4.5 Sudden Infant Death Syndrome (SIDS) (798.0)
4.6 Infant Sleep Apnea (770.80)
4.7 Congenital Central Hypoventilation Syndrome(770.81)
4.8 Sleeping Sickness (086)
4.9 Primary Snoring (780.53-1)
5. Sleep Disorders Associated with Metal Disorders
5.1 Psychoses (292-298)
5.2 Mood disorders (296-301)
5.3 Anxiety Disorders (300)
5.4 Panic disorders (300)
5.5 Alcoholism (303)
5.6 Post Traumatic Stress Disorder
5.7 Dissociative Disorders

*ICD-9 codes from the International Classification of Sleep Disorders in parenthesis.

IV. PROPOSED SLEEP DISORDERS
    a. Fragmentary Myoclonus (780.59-7)
    b. Sleep Hyperhydrosis(780.8)
    c. Menstrual Associated Sleep Disorder (780.54-3)
    d. Pregnancy-associated Sleep Disorder (780.59-6)
    e. Sleep-related neurogenic tachypnea (780.53-2)

SLEEP DISORDERS EVALUATION AND TREATMENT
    1. INSOMNIA (DIMS: Difficulty initiating and maintaining sleep):
       Evaluation, differential diagnosis and treatment.
    2. Sleep Hygiene Recommendations
    3. Medications that commonly cause insomnia

ERECTILE DISFUNCTION (ED) (780.56-3)

ENURESIS (780.56-0)

KLEIN-LEVINE SYNDROME (780.54-2)

CONFUSIONAL AROUSALS (307.46-2)

SLEEP TERRORS(307.46-1)

NIGHT SWEATS (Sleep Hyperhydrosis) (780.8):
    Definition and differential diagnosis.

EXCESIVE DAYTIME SLEEPINESS (EDS): Differential diagnosis

UPPER AIRWAY RESISTANCE SYNDROME

THERAPY FOR SLEEP DISORDERED BREATHING
    Snoring
    Surgery for OSA
    Oxygen
    Progesterone
    CPAP
    BiPAP
    CPAP COMPLIANCE
    SPLIT NIGHT STUDIES
    AutoCPAP
    Cheine-Stokes Breathing

UNIHEMISPHERIC SLEEP

*ICD-9 codes from the International Classification of Sleep Disorders in parenthesis.

SLEEP REGULATION
>   Suprachiasmatic Nucleus
>   Ultradian rhythm
>   Infradian rhythm
>   Circannual rhythm
>   Growth Hormone (GH)
>   Prolactin
>   Cortisol
>   TSH
>   LH
>   Melatonin
>   Tryptophan
>   Hypothyroidism
>   Neglect
>   Circadian rhythm and sleep

CHEMICALS AND SLEEP

SLEEP OTOGENY

NEWBORN EEG
>   Trace discontinue
>   Sleep Ontogeny in infancy
>   Beta-delta complexes
>   Theta burst
>   Frontal sharp waves
>   Difference in sleep and waking EEG
>   Alpha rhythm
>   Hypsarrhythmia

NORMAL SLEEP EEG
>   Alpha rhythm
>   1. Occipital alpha waves
>   2. Alpha wave frequency ontogeny
>   3. Distribution of alpha rhythm
>   4. Bilateral Symmetry
>   Mu rhythm
>   Beta activity
>   Theta activity
>   Sleep Onset
>   Stage I
>   Arousal
>   Sensory Threshold for arousal

*ICD-9 codes from the International Classification of Sleep Disorders in parenthesis.

EEG ACTIVITY OF SLEEP
> Vertex Sharp wave Transients
> K complexes and vertex transients
> Spindles
> Fast activity
> Positive occipital Sharp Transient (POST of sleep)
> Occipital Slow Transients)

SLEEP POLYSOMNOGRAPHY (PSG)
> SUMMARY OF SLEEP PSG SCORING
> Wake
> RAPID EYE MOVEMENT (REM)
> Stage I
> Stage II
> Stage III
> Stage IV
> Movement time
> Awakening
> Arousal
> PLM's
> Movement Associated Arousal
> Movement Index
> Movement-Arousal Index (MAI)
> Sleep Onset Latency
> REM latency

ATYPICAL SLEEP PATTERNS
> 1. alpha-Delta sleep
> 2. REM spindle
> 3. SLEEP ONSET REM (SOREM)
> 4. REM without atonia
> Awakening in MSLT
> Narcolepsy
> REM
> Obstructive apnea
> Mixed apnea
> Central apnea
> Arousals
> PSG PEARLS

CYCLICAL VARIATION OF HEART RATE (CVHR)

AROUSALS

OSA ARRYTHMIAS

*ICD-9 codes from the International Classification of Sleep Disorders in parenthesis.

GERD

DECREASED REM LATENCY

MULTIPLE SLEEP LATENCY TEST (MSLT)

MAINTENANCE OF WAKEFULNESS TEST (MWT)

MOOD DISORDERS AND PSG FINDINGS
    PSG
    Decreased REM density causes
    Endogenous depression
    Antidepressant treatment of major depression

ANXIETY DISORDERS
    Panic Disorder
    Obsessive-compulsive Disorders
    Phobia
    Generalized anxiety disorder
    Posttraumatic Stress Disorder (PTSD)
    PSG findings in anxiety disorders
    Differential diagnosis of insomnia secondary to anxiety disorders
        1. Psycho physiologic insomnia
        2. Major Depression
        3. Organic causes
        4. Nocturnal panic attacks
    Treatment of anxiety disorders

SCHIZOPHRENIA
    1. Diagnostic criteria
    2. PSG findings

DEMENTIA
    PSG Findings
    COMA
    PSG findings

EFFECTS OF MEDICATIONS ON SLEEP AND WAKEFULNESS
    Hypnotics: Ultra rapid elimination, rapid elimination, relative
    rapid elimination, slow elimination, slow absorption.
    Antidepressants: sedating, less side effects, increased psychomotor
    and cognitive function.
    Lithium
    Neuroleptics

*ICD-9 codes from the International Classification of Sleep Disorders in parenthesis.

Stimulants
Anticonvulsivants
Antiemetics
Tricyclics
Heterocyclic Antidepressants-second generation
Selective serotonin reuptake inhibitors
Barbiturics
Benzodiazepines
Marihuana
Morphine
Hyperthyroidism

ANTYPSYCHOTICS GROUPS BY SIDE EFFECTS

INDICATIONS FOR CARDIOPULMONARY SLEEP TESTING (POLYSOMNOGRAPHY (PSG))

EFFECTS OF MEDICATIONS ON SLEEP AND WAKEFULNESS
Hypnotics
1. Ultra rapid elimination
2. Rapid elimination
3. Relative Rapid Elimination
4. Slow Elimination
5. Slow Absorption

Antidepressants (AD)
1. Sedating
2. Less side effects
3. Increase Psychomotor and cognitive function

Lithium
Narcoleptics
Stimulants
Anticonvulsivants
Antiemetics
Tryciclics
Heterocyclic AD of second generation
Selective Serotonin Reuptake Inhibitors (SSRI's)
Barbiturics
Benzodiazepines
Marihuana
Morphine
Hyperthyroidism

ANTIPSYCHOTIC GROUPS BY SIDE EFFECTS

Indications of sleep cardiopulmonary (Polysomnography) testing

*ICD-9 codes from the International Classification of Sleep Disorders in parenthesis.

Tables
1. Differential Diagnosis of Dificulty Initiating Sleep complaint.
2. Drugs that commonly cause Insomnia

Sample of Sleep Diary.
Sample Sleep Study Order Form-Sleep ePortal Sleep Disorders Center.
Aknowledgements.

*ICD-9 codes from the International Classification of Sleep Disorders in parenthesis.

SLEEP DISORDERS CLASSIFICATION

Sleep disorders are classified in four general groups:

I. Parasomnias: or "things that go bump in the night"
II. Dissomnias: Intrinsic, Extrinsic sleep disorders and circadian sleep disorders
III. Medical/Psychiatric sleep Disorders
IV. Proposed Sleep Disorders

I. PARASOMNIAS*

1. Non-REM Parasomnias

1.1 Disorders of Arousals
- Confusional Arousals (307.46-2)
- Sleepwalking (307.46-0)
- Sleep Terror (307.46.1)
- Sleep-Related eating (780.52-8)

Evaluate if:
- Potential for harm to self (Injurious behavior)
- Potential for harm to others (violent behavior)
- Severe disruption of other household members
- Resultant excessive daytime sleepiness (EDS)
- Atypical clinical features

Treatment:
- None (most)
- Improve sleep hygiene
- Benzodiazepines
- Tricyclic Antidepressants (TCA)
- Hypnosis

2. Primary Miscellaneous Sleep phenomena (Sleep Stage)
- Bruxism (1, 2, REM) (306.8): Teeth grinding. Clinically the patient may wake up with jaw pain and if severe may have abnormal wear of teeth. The most common cause is inadequate alignment of teeth so orthodontic referral is required. An oral appliance may help protect the teeth.
- Enuresis (Any) (780.56-0) (page 17)
- Rhythmic Movement Disorder (Any) (307.3)
- Periodic Leg Movement (PLM) Disorder (780.52.4)
- Somniloquy (Sleep Talking) (1,2, REM) (307. 47-3)

3. REM Parasomnias

*ICD-9 codes from the International Classification of Sleep Disorders in parenthesis.

3.1. Sinus Arrest (780.56-8)
Sinus arrest of more than 2.5 seconds that occurs during REM sleep, is not related to any other sleep complaint and is not due to any other cardiac or sleep disorder that has been associated with cardiac irregularities such as the Obstructive Sleep Apnea Syndrome. Treatment consists of cardiology referral for permanent pacemaker placement.

3.2. REM behavior disorder (RBD) (780.59-0)
- Intermittent loss of REM atonia
- Elaborate motor activity
- Dream mentation
- Elderly
- Reduced Striatal Dopamine Activity
- Neurological disorders
- Associated with other sleep disorders
  Narcolepsy
  OSA
- RBD etiology
  - o Idiopathic 42%
  - o Neurologic: 57%
    - Alpha synucleinopathies (most Neurologic causes): Parkinson's, Dementia with Lewy Bodies, Multiple System Atrophy
    - Vascular
    - Toxic/metabolic
    - Tumor
    - Infectious, post-infectious
    - Degenerative
    - Traumatic
    - Developmental/congenital/familial
    - Narcolepsy (8%)
    - Idiopathic
  - o Psychiatric: 9%
    - Adjustment disorder (divorce, MVA)
    - Chronic abstinence
    - Fluoxetine rx of OCD
    - Rapid imipramine withdrawal
  - o Endocrine 1%
- RBD clinical forms
  - o Acute
    - Withdrawal: Alcohol, barbiturates
    - Intoxication: TCA's, SSRI's, Venlafaxine, Mirtazapine.
  - o Chronic
- RBD presenting complaints:
  - o Sleep injury 80%

*ICD-9 codes from the International Classification of Sleep Disorders in parenthesis.

- o Sleep disruption 20%
- o Altered dreams 87%
- o Dream enacting behavior 87%
- o Increased %SWS sleep 80%
- o Periodic NREM leg movements 61%
- o Aperiodic NREM leg movements 37%
- o Response to clonazepam 90%
- ❑ Age of presentation
  - o Age= 61 years old (36-84)
  - o Male 87%
  - o Prodrome 25%
- ❑ Psychiatric evaluation
  - o Interview
  - o Psychometric testing
- ❑ Neurologic
  - o Clinical exam, EEG
  - o CT, MRI of brain
  - o Polysomnography (PSG) full seizure montage
  - o Paper speed at least 15mm/sec
  - o Cont. a/v monitoring
- ❑ Dx criteria:
  - o Either:
  - o A history of problematic motor ax. During sleep
  - o Or observed integrated motor ax during sleep
  - o And intermittent or persistent EMG augmentation during REM sleep (loss of atonia)
  - o RBD PSG Findings: increased phasic or tonic REM EMG (97%), ambiguous sleep (3%), abnormal gross motor behavior (30%), OSA (34%), PLMS more than 20/h (47%), mean % REM sleep=17%, Mean % SWS=12.5%. Fewer PLMS arousals and higher PLM index in REM sleep, in RBD than in Restless Legs Syndrome (RLS)
- ❑ RBD diff dx:
  - o Nocturnal seizures
  - o Disorders of arousal
  - o Nocturnal panic disorder
  - o Post Traumatic Stress Disorder (PTSD)
  - o Overlap syndrome
  - o Psychogenic dissociative disorder
  - o Malingering
- ❑ There is a higher incidence of RBD in narcoleptics
- ❑ Parkinsonism may emerge together or RBD before Parkinsonism (mean 13 years)
- ❑ RBD may herald the onset of Parkinsonism or Shy-Dragger by up to 15 years
- ❑ RBD tx:
  - o Clonazepam: 0.75-1.25 mg (.25-3mg) for 2.5y (0.5-9years)
    - • Serotonergic

*ICD-9 codes from the International Classification of Sleep Disorders in parenthesis.

- GABAergic
- DA antagonist
- Anticonvulsant
- Side effects: sedation, cognitive effects, gait unsteadiness, impotence. Caution in OSA, autonomic instability, dementia, gait disturbances.
  - o Other benzodiazepines
  - o Quetiapine
  - o Melatonin: 3-12 mg, effective in most patients in few trials.
  - o Pramipexole: 0.5-1 mg, limited data indicates effectiveness in most patients.
  - o Bedroom safety.

3.1 Nightmares (307.47-0) Frightening dreams that awaken the patient from sleep.

3.2 Sleep paralysis (780.56-2) Upon sleep onset or awakening there is inability to move. PSG reveals REM onset sleep. It may be familial or associated with narcolepsy.

3.3 Impaired sleep-related penile erections (780.56-3) See Erectile Dysfunction.

3.4 Sleep related painful erections (780.56-4) Pain during nocturnal erections not associated with organic causes. During daytime erections there is no pain. PSG reveals penile erections associated with awakening from REM sleep.

4. SLEEP-WAKE TRANSITION DISORDERS

4.1 Rhythmic Movement Disorder (307.3) Stereotyped, repetitive movements involving large muscle groups. They may present as head banging, head rolling, body rocking or body rolling. They occur during sleep onset and are carried into light sleep. Onset is during the first 2 years of life.

4.2 Sleep Starts (307.47-2) At sleep onset there are sudden and brief contractions of legs, arms or head. They are associated with a feeling of falling, a sensory flash or a hypnagogic dream (dream while falling asleep). When severe they may lead to insomnia.

4.3 Sleep Talking (307.47-3) Episodes of speech or utterances without recall for the event. May be associated with febrile illness or with another sleep disorder such as REM sleep behavior disorder, sleep walking or obstructive sleep apnea.

4.4 Nocturnal Leg Cramps (729.82) Foot or calf painful tension sensation during sleep not associated with an underlying medical condition. They resolve with local massage or heat and disrupt sleep.

II. DYSOMNIAS

II.1 Intrinsic
II.1.1 Psycho physiologic insomnia (307.42-0)
- o Sleep Latency > 30 min.
- o TST < 6.5 hours
II.1.2 Sleep state misperception (307.49-1)
- o Sleep Latency < 15-20 min.

*ICD-9 codes from the International Classification of Sleep Disorders in parenthesis.

- o MSLT sleep Lat > 10 min.
- o TST >= 6.5 hours.

II.1.3 Idiopathic insomnia (780.52-7)
II.1.4 Narcolepsy (347)
- ❑ Most cases sporadic but there is evidence suggesting genetic factors. Most human cases are probably caused by an autoimmune-mediated destruction of hypocretin neurons, resulting in undetectable or rarely elevated levels of hypocretin-1 levels in the CSF.   HLA-DR2 and HLA-DQB1*0602 positivity have been associated with Narcolepsy-cataplexy.
- ❑ Secondary or Symptomatic narcolepsy: Hypothalamic pathologies (Acute Disseminated encephalomyelitis, Multiple Sclerosis, Midbrain glioblastoma, Cerebral sarcoidosis, Pontine infarcts, Hypothalamic syndrome, Craniopharyngioma, Third ventricle tumors, Pituitary Adenoma), Niemann Pick Disease Type C, Pradder Willi Syndrome, Coffin-Lowry syndrome, Late onset Congenital Hypoventilation Syndrome and Myotonic Dystrophy.
- ❑ Narcolepsy symptoms

Primary:
- o EDS and irresistible sleep episodes (first)
- o Cataplexy (usually with above but may occur 20 years later, never or rarely before)

Secondary
- o Hypnagogic hallucinations
- o Sleep paralysis
- o Automatic behavior
- o Disrupted nocturnal sleep
- ❑ Onset during adolescence, but may present even before 5 years of age.
- ❑ Cataplexy may or may not be present at onset or during course. Cataplexy is rare before 5 years of age.
- ❑ Secondary symptoms appear in later decades
- ❑ MSLT criteria:

Diagnostic
Mean Sleep Latency less of equal to 5 or 8 minutes
REM sleep on 2 naps: SOREM'S (REM lat <15 min).
Suggestive:
Mean latency 5-10 minutes
REM onset sleep on one nap
Differential features with idiopathic hypersomnia: absence of SOREM's on MSLT, extended sleep time and no REM-related symptoms.
- ❑ MSLT not infallible
- ❑ Cataplexy and sleep paralysis treatment
  - o Nonatropinic tricyclics are best:
  - o Viloxazine HCL (50mg tablets) Normal dose 150-200mg qd
  - o Fluoxetine HCL (20 mg) Nl: 1 qd in am
  - o Clomipramine (25-50 mg tablets) 75-125 mg qhs.

*ICD-9 codes from the International Classification of Sleep Disorders in parenthesis.

❑ Treatment of sleepiness
Behavioral:
- o Scheduled short 15 min daytime naps
- o Best time: 10:30AM, 1PM, 4 PM

Nutrition:
- o Avoid heavy lunches
- o Avoid alcohol
- o Avoid chocolate and other substances with paradoxical effects

Medication:
Children & adolescents:
- o Pemoline (18.75 and 37.5 mg tablets): increase weekly up to 37-150mg/d
- o Modafinil: first choice. Low abuse potential

Adults:
- o Methylphenidate (5mg) 30-45 min AC of PC (empty stomach). Repeat doses PRN and avoid large doses. Usual: 20-40mg/d.
- o Slow-release form 20mg q am.
- o Pemoline (37.5mg): 100-150mg/d. One-two daily doses, am and at noon.
- o Dexedrine (5mg) 4-8mg/d in two doses
- o Modafinil (Provigil): a nonamphetamine stimulant of low abuse potential. First line agent for EDS in narcolepsy, residual EDS in treated OSA and in shift workers. Women usually need 100mg/d. In general range is between 200 and 400 mg/d. A dose of 400 mg is equivalent to 600 mg of caffeine as alertness promoting in sleep deprived subjects. Precautions: LVH, ischemic ECG changes, chest pain, arrhythmia or other significant manifestations of mitral valve prolapse associated with CNS stimulants. Recent MI or unstable angina. History of psychosis, severe renal impairment or severe hepatic impairment. Monitor BP. No data available of effects in hypertensive patients.
- o Treatment of disturbed nocturnal sleep: GABA.

SOREM ON MSLT: REM lat < 20 min.
- o Sedative withdrawal
- o Narcolepsy
- o Infancy
- o Time Zone shifts
- o Sleep Deprivation

II.1.5 Idiopathic hypersomnia (780.54-7): Increased Total Sleep Time, Short sleep latency, no SOREM's in MSLT.
II.1.6 Recurrent hypersomnia (780.54-2)
II.1.7 Posttraumatic hypersomnia (780.54-8)
II.1.8 Obstructive Sleep Apnea (OSA) (780.53-0)
Pediatrics: Indications for PSG in children for OSA/Obesity Hypoventilation (OHV)
❑ Differentiate benign snoring from OSA/OHV
❑ Snoring and:

*ICD-9 codes from the International Classification of Sleep Disorders in parenthesis.

- o Unexplained disturbed sleep pattern
- o Excessive Daytime Sleepiness (EDS)
- o Cor Pulmonale
- o Failure to thrive
- o Polycythemia
- o CHF
- o ADHD and related behaviors
- ❏ Formal PSG may be used to identify children at high risk for postoperative upper airway obstruction following tonsillectomy & adenectomy (T&A)
- ❏ Also in a child with laryngomalacia whose symptoms are worse asleep than awake and/or has failure to thrive (FTT) or Cor Pulmonale
  - o Symptoms worst asleep &/or
  - o FTT &/or
  - o Cor Pulmonale
- ❏ Obese child with:
  - o Snoring
  - o EDS
  - o Disturbed sleep
  - o CHF
  - o Polycythemia or
  - o Cor Pulmonale
- ❏ In children with any condition that interacts and may be exacerbated by OSA/OHV who have unexplained snoring and:
  - o FTT
  - o Cor Pulmonale
  - o Polycythemia
  - o CHF
- ❏ PSG norms during childhood
  - o Total Sleep Time (TST) 560 minutes=9.3 hours
  - o Sleep efficiency=99%
  - o Latency to stage 1=12 min
  - o Latency to stage 2= 16 min
  - o % of stage1=7%
  - o Stage 2=44%
  - o Stage 3=10%
  - o Stage 4=19%
  - o REM=20%
  - o REM latency= 160 minutes=2.66 hours (70-100min young adults, up to 120 min adults)
  - o MSLT REM latency= 17-18 minutes
  - o Apnea index=1-2/hour (Adults more than 10)
    - ❏ PSG during lab conditions:
  - o TST= >=5 hours
  - o Sleep efficiency=>=85%
  - o REM sleep= 15-30% of TST

*ICD-9 codes from the International Classification of Sleep Disorders in parenthesis.

- o SWS= 10-40% of TST
- o Apnea index (AI)=<=1/h
- o Peak pCO2=<=53mmHg
- o Change in pCO2=<=13
- o Duration of hypoventilation (pCO2>45mmHg)=<=60%TST
- o SaO2 nadir= >=92%
- o Desaturation >=4%=<=1.4/h
- o Change in SaO2= <=8%

OSA in adults: studies of the prevalence of sleep disordered breathing have reported that 24% of men and 9% of women ages 30-60 have mild OSA (Apnea Hypopnea Index (AHI):5-15 events per hour) and 9% of men and 4% of women have moderate OSA (AHI:15-30). In general, OSA with daytime impairment or the sleep apnea syndrome is estimated to occur in one out of 20 adults and asymptomatic OSA occurs in one out of five adults. When body mass index (BMI) is taken into consideration to estimate the prevalence of OSA, in general adult women and men with a BMI of 25-28, roughly 1 out of 5 has at least mild OSA and 1 out 15 has moderate OSA.

The complications of obstructive sleep apnea range from behavioral complications (irritability, depression), hypertension, cardiovascular and cerebrovascular morbidity and mortality, motor vehicle and occupational accidents and decreased quality of life.

Severe sleep apnea is a risk factor for increased motor vehicle accidents. CPAP treatment seems to normalize crash risk in this high-risk group. The effects of sleep duration of less than 5 hours are comparable to the effects on performance from severe OSA in commercial drivers. The correlation between mild to moderate sleep apnea with the incidence of motor vehicle accidents is less clear.
High risk drivers are defined by one of the following: a recent fall-asleep crash, repeated "near miss" fall-asleep episodes while driving, repeatedly falling asleep in other active situations (during conversations or at meal table), very high score on Epworth Sleepiness Scale (more than 15?, such score is not defined). The Multiple Wake Latency Test is not helpful to predict crash risk.

The ATS guidelines recommend categorical reporting of sleep apnea in drivers (does no include commercial drivers) if they had a previous crash due to falling asleep and if the individual refuses treatment. Of note is that REM related OSA has not been correlated with increased daytime sleepiness as measured by MSLT. (Sleep, Vol.25, No. 3, 2002). We could infer that REM related OSA is excluded from the increased risk in crashes.

A practical approach to address the medico-legal risk in drivers is to document warning patient of risk (key step), to recommend to stop driving until study/treatment to high-risk patients and to make a study available within days to avoid excessive loss of workdays. Every state has different viewpoints on sleepiness during driving. It is legally prudent not to report without patient written permission and to know your state laws and consult with a lawyer prior to reporting.

*ICD-9 codes from the International Classification of Sleep Disorders in parenthesis.

Sleep apnea is correlated with body mass index. A reduction in 20% of base line weight has been correlated with a reduction in the AHI by 50%. Potentially modifiable risk factors that have been linked to OSA include overweight and obesity, smoking, alcohol, nasal congestion and estrogen depletion in menopause. So far the only proven risk factor is obesity, so the primary care physician plays a pivotal role in the prevention and management of OSA.

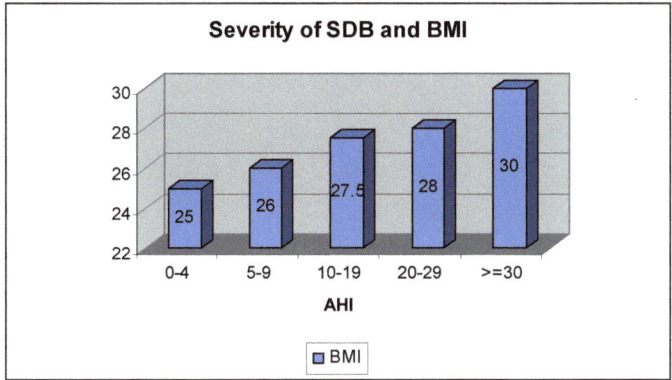

*SDB=Sleep Disordered Breathing. BMI: Body mass index. AJRCCM-Young, et al. May, 2002.

*ICD-9 codes from the International Classification of Sleep Disorders in parenthesis.

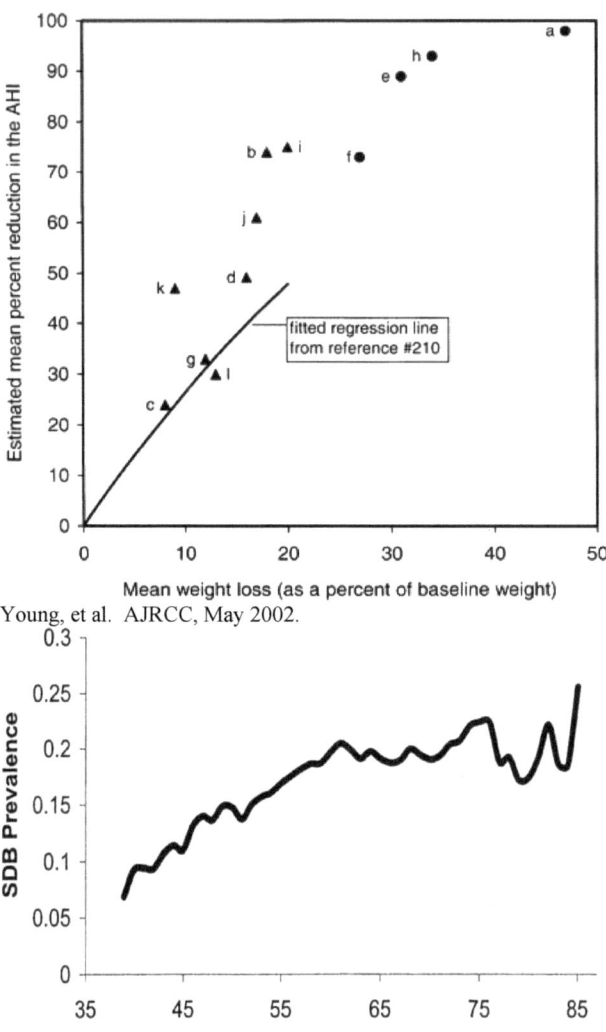

Young, et al. AJRCC, May 2002.

Prevalence of Sleep Disordered Breathing with age. Young et al. AJRCCM, May 2002.

*ICD-9 codes from the International Classification of Sleep Disorders in parenthesis.

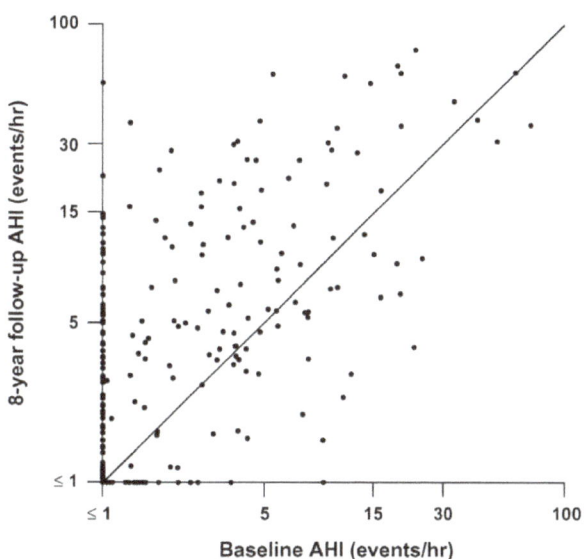

Progression of OSA with time is likely in patients with habitual snoring, increasing BMI, and in older patients. The Wisconsin Sleep Cohort Study. Young, et al. AJRCCM, May 2002.

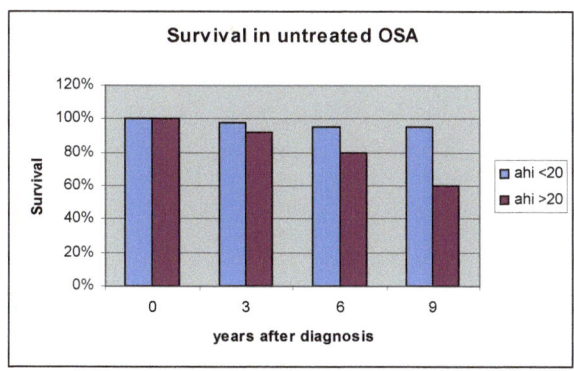

*ICD-9 codes from the International Classification of Sleep Disorders in parenthesis.

Mortality and apnea index in OSA. Chest 1988; 94:9-14.

II.1.9   Central sleep apnea syndrome (780.51-0): central apneas (complete cessation of airflow and respiratory effort) associated with sleep disruption or oxygen Desaturation. There is reduced mean sleep latency on the MSLT(less than 10 minutes) and it may be associated with obstructive sleep apnea and other sleep disorders. There may be Brady tachycardia. The patient may complain of difficulty initiating or maintaining sleep or excessive sleepiness.

II.1.10   Central alveolar hypoventilation syndrome (780.51-1): Hypoventilation that leads to oxygen Desaturation and that is worsened during sleep. The patient complains of insomnia or sleepiness. There is absence of primary pulmonary conditions, peripheral neuromuscular disorders or skeletal malformations affecting ventilation. It may be associated with other neurological disorders affecting the CNS control of breathing. Other sleep disorders may be associated. On PSG there will be hypopneas with arousals and desaturations. The MSLT will have also a mean sleep latency of less than 190 minutes.

II.1.11   Periodic Limb movement disorder (PLMD) (780.52-4) Repetitive, highly stereotyped limb movements associated some times with sleep disruption. The may disturb the sleep of the bed partner as well. It may be related to a medication side effect or withdrawal.

II.1.12   Restless legs syndrome (RLS) (780.52-5) Creeping legs sensation that lead to an irresistible urge to move the legs occurring at sleep onset. It may be associated with PLMD. Antidepressants (except wellbutrin) and antiemetics exacerbate RLS.

- ❑ **TX for PLMD & RLS**
- ❑ Hypnoptics such as Clonazepam 0.5-4 mg/d (0.5, 1 and 2 mg): reduces PLMs and arousals (may get nasty syndrome). Restoril and Ambien. Gabapentin has been used with success.
- ❑ Darvocet N-100 to decrease arousals
- ❑ Tylenol #3
- ❑ Tylenol with oxycodone 5mg, decreases PLMs & arousals
- ❑ Last 3 opioids 1-3 tabs a day some times more
- ❑ Methadone 5-20 mg qd for more severe cases
- ❑ Watch constipation and addiction/tolerance
- ❑ Baclofen 10, 20mg, 20-40 mg most effective (10-120mg) decreases arousals, decreases PLM's amplitude. Side effects: Drowsiness, dizziness, fatigue.
- ❑ Carbamazepine 100, 200 mg range 200-600mg or more. Monitor CBC (leucopenia), LFT's, BUN creatinine, tegretol level, drowsiness, ataxia.
- ❑ Adrenergic agents:
  - ○ Clonidine 0.1-0.9mg/d to decrease leg sensations
  - ○ Phenoxybenzamine (alfa blocker) 10-20 mg/d

Dose for all drugs three divided doses, one 2 hours prior to HS and at hs and in the middle of the night PRN. May use daytime dose in needed.
DA agonists, opioids and benzodiazepines for RLS and PLMs.

*ICD-9 codes from the International Classification of Sleep Disorders in parenthesis.

Clonidine and Tegretol for RLS, Baclofen for PLMS.
TCA's associated with RBD's and PLM's.

II.2 Intrinsic sleep disorder NOS

II.3 Extrinsic

- **Inadequate sleep hygiene (307.41-1)** Insomnia or sleepiness resulting from inadequate habits not conducive to sleep. Refer to Sleep Hygiene Recommendations on page on page 15.
- **Environmental sleep disorder (780.52-6)** Sleep is disrupted due to environmental factors such as room temperature, noise and the like.
- **Altitude insomnia (289.0)** Reduced sleep time, decreased sleep efficiency, increased sleep latency, increased arousal index and wake time typically occurring after a temporary ascent to more than 4000 meters. Periodic breathing and oxygen desaturation during sleep. Insomnia complaint not caused by another sleep or psychiatric disorder.
- **Adjustment sleep disorder (307.41-0)** A complaint of insomnia or excessive daytime sleepiness related to an acute stressor.
- **Insufficient sleep syndrome (307.49-4)** The patient voluntarily sleeps less than the amount of time expected for his age. There is a complaint of excessive daytime sleepiness or difficulty initiating sleep. Sleep efficiency is greater than 85% and sleep latency less than 15 minutes on PSG and MSLT that demonstrates excessive sleepiness. Treatment is to institute a longer sleep episode.
- **Limit-setting sleep disorder (307.42-4)** Occurs typically in children were caregivers fail to set a regular bedtime. The child refuses to go to bed at a reasonable time. Establishing a routine that leads to sleep such as a bath before bedtime and reading a story at bedtime may help solve the problem.
- **Sleep-onset association disorder (307.42-5)** It is the failure to fall asleep in the absence of a specific object or set of circumstances such as music, television watching, nursing or other.
- **Food allergy insomnia (780.52-2)** Sleep disturbance related to the introduction of a particular food or drink with restoration of normal sleep pattern within 4 weeks of withdrawal of the allergen. In children older than 3 years other symptoms of allergy may appear such as skin rash, gastrointestinal upset, lethargy, psychomotor agitation and respiratory difficulties. There are raised antibodies to the causative agent. PSG demonstrates frequent arousals.
- **Nocturnal eating (drinking) syndrome (780.52-8)** The patient complains of difficulty maintaining sleep with frequent awakenings to eat or drink, followed by normal sleep onset. There is absence of any other sleep, psychiatric or medical disorder such as hypoglycemia or bulimia to account for the sleep complaint. PSG reveals increased number and duration of arousals.

*ICD-9 codes from the International Classification of Sleep Disorders in parenthesis.

- **Hypnotic-dependent sleep disorder (780.52-8)** Following at least 3 weeks of nearly daily hypnoptic use, the patient complaints of insomnia or excessive daytime sleepiness due to tolerance or withdrawal from such medications.
- **Stimulant-dependent sleep disorder (780.52-1)** Insomnia or excessive daytime sleepiness temporarily related to the use or withdrawal of stimulants. May be associated with abuse or dependence of the stimulant.
- **Alcohol-dependent sleep disorder (780.52-3)** The need to drink alcohol for at least one month to induce sleep.
- **Toxin-induced sleep disorder (780.54-6)** Poisoning with heavy metals or organic toxins leads to either excessive daytime sleepiness or insomnia.
- **Extrinsic sleep disorder NOS**

II.4 Circadian rhythm sleep disorders

- **Time zone change (jet lag) syndrome (307.45-0)** Multiple somatic complaints that occur after traveling through multiple time zones associated with difficulty initiating or maintaining sleep, excessive sleepiness, decreased alertness and performance.
- **Shift work sleep disorder (307.45-1)** Work schedule outside of conventional sleep-wake cycle leading to insomnia or sleepiness. Maintaining a regular work schedule helps to consolidate sleep at the same time every day. A one or two hour difference in sleep time during off days should be maintained to avoid sleep disturbances.
- **Irregular sleep-wake pattern (307.45-3)** It is the absence of a regular sleep period over 24 hours. There is loss of temperature pattern for at least 24 hours or loss of normal sleep-wake pattern demonstrated by 24 hour PSG. The total 24-hour sleep time is normal for age. When due to environmental or social factors (extrinsic) or due to abnormal circadian pacemaker (intrinsic).
- **Delayed sleep phase syndrome (780.55-0)** There is a delay in the sleep period with resultant difficulty waking up at a desired time and excessive daytime sleepiness. It may be intrinsic or extrinsic.
- **Advanced sleep phase syndrome (780.55-1)** Sleep is initiated at an earlier than desired clock time with resultant awakening at an earlier time. This syndrome is common in the elderly and may lead to social isolation.
- **Non-24 hour sleep-wake disorder (780.55-2)** A chronic 1-2 hour delay in sleep time with a progressive delay in 24 hour temperature nadir over 24 hour monitoring.
- **Circadian rhythm sleep disorder NOS**

III. Secondary Sleep Phenomena
1. Neurological
1.1. Primary Headache
- Migraine
- Cluster
- Chronic paroxysmal hemi crania

*ICD-9 codes from the International Classification of Sleep Disorders in parenthesis.

- Hypnic headache
- Exploding head syndrome

1.2. Secondary Headache
- Sleep-disordered Breathing
1.3. Fatal familial insomnia (337.9)
- Difficulty Initiating Sleep (DIS)
- Within months progresses to total lack of sleep
- Later to spontaneous lapses from quiet wakefulness into a sleep state with enacted dreams (oneiric stupor)
- Associated with thalamic degeneration
- Death
1.4 Sleep-related epilepsy (345)
- Any phenomenon that is recurrent, stereotyped and inappropriate may represent a seizure
- Conventional seizures: 10% will have these spells exclusively during sleep.
- Unconventional:
  - Episodic nocturnal wandering
    - Episodic nocturnal wandering
    - Same than sleepwalking or sleep terrors: screaming, vocalizations, violent automatism
    - Amnesic for spell, self-injury
    - No hx of sz.
  - Hypnogenic paroxysmal Dystonia
  - Tonic spasms and violent movements during sleep-vocalizations, laughter
  - Nocturnal often multiple
  - Rare diurnal
  - During NREM, often after an "arousal"
  - No EEG abnormalities during or between spells
  - No post-ictal period- either clinical or EEG
  - Frontal lobe seizures
  - May occur in clusters (50/d) with sz-free intervals of months
  - Nocturnal
  - EEG may show focal abnormality, a vertex wave followed by generalized suppression, then artifact. But it may be normal even during clinical attack.
  - Bizarre behavior:
    - Uncontrollable running, yelling
    - Vehement cursing, groaning, struggling
    - Foot-stomping, kicking
    - Screaming with acute panic
  - Hallucinations- visual, auditory, olfactory

*ICD-9 codes from the International Classification of Sleep Disorders in parenthesis.

- o May retain some degree of consciousness, ability to follows simple commands.
- o Sub cortical seizures

- o Motor manifestations:
    - Tonic axial
    - Tonic axo-rhizomelic
    - Global tonic
    - Asymmetric tonic
    - Unilateral tonic (hemi-tonic)
- o Vegetative phenomena
    - Respiratory: polypnea, apnea, cry
    - CVS: tachycardia, HTN
    - Mydriasis
    - Vasomotor: red face, piloerection, lacrimation, salivation, hyper/hypo-thermia
- o Psychic phenomena
    - Loss or clouding of consciousness
    - Rapid return to consciousness
- o EEG correlates
    - Desynchronization
    - Hyper synchronization
    - Desynchronization >hyper synchronization
    - Recruiting rhythm (10 Hz)
    - A given pt. May have identical clinical seizure with different EEG pattern.
    - Immediate return to pre-ictal pattern
- o Refractory to anticonvulsants
- o Reported effective
    - Methylphenidate
    - Bromocryptine/morphine
    - Clonidine, total sympathectomy.
- o Seizures as isolated arousals
- o Paroxysmal epileptic discharges during NREM resulting in arousal without other symptoms.
- o Present as diurnal hypersomnia
- o No hx of seizures
- o No waking EEG abnormality.
- o TX: Anticonvulsants or sedative/hypnotics
- o Seizures as "recurrent nightmares"
- o "Nightmares" as only manifestation.
- o May occur during either REM or NREM sleep
- o Electrical status Epilepticus of sleep
- o Continuous slow spike and SW ax during sleep

*ICD-9 codes from the International Classification of Sleep Disorders in parenthesis.

- Clinically may have sx, psychomotor retardation or asymptomatic
- Isolated unusual symptoms
- Chest pain/arrhythmias
- Stridor/laryngospasm
- Apnea
- Flushing/pallor
- Diaphoretic/piloerection
- Emesis
- Coughing
- Sexual automatism
- Headache
- Pain

1.5 Electrical Status Epilepticus of Sleep (345.8)
- Pure NREM association
- Continuous and diffuse spike-SW complexes through NREM

1.6 Cerebral degenerative disorders

1.7 Dementia (331)

1.8 Parkinsonism (332-333)

2. Cardio-Pulmonary Sleep Phenomena
- Arrhythmias:
  Sinus Arrest: Asystole in REM sleep (5-9 sec) Tx: Permanent Pacemaker.
  Noise induced arousal with syncope and urine incontinence
- Angina: Nocturnal cardiac ischemia (may be asymptomatic) (411-414)
- Asthma/COPD (490-494)
- Sleep related Asthma (493)
- Abnormal swallowing
  Coughing
  Aspiration
  Choking
- Sleep-related laryingospasm
- Primary snoring

3. G-I
- Reflux (530.1)
- Diffuse esophageal spasm
  Mimics nocturnal cardiac disease with or without arrhythmias

4. Miscellaneous

4.1 Nocturnal Muscle Cramps
- Tx: quinine or verapamil
- Sx of underlying NMS disease
  Muscular dystrophies
  Amyotrophic Lateral Sclerosis
- Common complaint in

*ICD-9 codes from the International Classification of Sleep Disorders in parenthesis.

Periodic Leg Movement disorder (PLM)
Restless Leg Syndrome (RLS)

4.2 Nocturnal Paroxysmal Dystonia (NPD) (780.59-1) Dystonic or dyskinetic episodes lasting 15-60 seconds to 60 minutes repeated during NREM sleep.

4.3 Sudden unexplained nocturnal death syndrome (SUDS) (780.59-3) Sudden cardiopulmonary arrest during sleep in otherwise healthy adults particularly of South Asian descent.

4.4 Benign neonatal sleep myoclonus (780.59-5) Asynchronous brief (40-300 milliseconds) jerks or the limbs or trunk during quiet sleep not associated with an underlying medical condition that could explain the symptoms.

4.5 Sudden Infant Death Syndrome (SIDS) (798.0) Unexpected infant (less than 12 months of age) death, occurring usually during sleep, unexplained at autopsy. It is rare in children between 12 and 24 months of age.

4.6 Infant Sleep Apnea (770.80) Central apneas greater than 20 seconds or obstructive apneas greater than 10 seconds. It may be associated with bradycardia, cyanosis, oxygen desaturations below 85%, hypercapnia ($pCO2 > 45$), color change (pallor or cyanosis), tone change (limpness, rarely stiffness) or noisy breathing during sleep. An identifiable cause may be found.

4.7 Congenital Central Hypoventilation Syndrome (770.81) Hypoventilation worse during sleep and not explained by primary pulmonary disorder or muscle weakness.

4.8 Sleeping sickness (086) Trypanosomiasis causing chronic meningoencephalomyelitis leading to severe sleepiness

4.9 Primary Snoring (780.53-1) snoring documented by observer or by PSG not associated with insomnia or excessive daytime sleepiness, oxygen desaturations, arousals or cardiac disturbances. Respiratory and sleep patterns are normal.

5. **Sleep Disorders associated with mental Disorders**
   5.1 Psychoses (292-298)
   5.2 Mood Disorders (296-301)
   5.3 Anxiety Disorders (300)
   5.4 Panic Disorders (300)
       Nocturnal Panic
       o Usually with Daytime panic
       o   Exclusively during sleep period
       Symptom overlap with other parasomnias
   5.5 Alcoholism (303)
   5.6 Post Traumatic Stress disorder (PTSD)
       o Bad dreams (54%)
       o Intrusive thoughts and images while trying to sleep
       o "Dreams" from any state
       o Broken REM atonia (may be present)
       o Re-experience of trauma
       o Recurrent intrusive recollections
       o Acting out or feeling as if the traumatic event were recurring

*ICD-9 codes from the International Classification of Sleep Disorders in parenthesis.

    o Social numbness or withdrawal

5.7 Dissociative Disorders
- o Bizarre and potentially injurious
- o May arise predominately or exclusively from the sleep period
  PSG: behaviors arising from well-developed wakefulness

IV   Proposed Sleep Disorders
  - **a. Fragmentary myoclonus (780.59-7)**
    - ❑ EDS
    - ❑ Frequent Brief myoclonic jerks
    - ❑ NREM at random
    - ❑ Many muscle groups
  - **b. Sleep Hyperhydrosis (780.8)**
    - ❑ Rare idiopathic
    - ❑ Usually underlying disease
  - **c. Menstrual Associated sleep disorder (780.54-3)** Insomnia or excessive daytime sleepiness of at least 3 months duration, temporally correlated with the menstrual cycle or insomnia associated with menopause.
  - **d. Pregnancy-associated sleep disorder (780.59-6)** Insomnia or excessive daytime sleepiness during pregnancy.
  - **e. Sleep-related neurogenic tachypnea (780.53-2)**
    - ❑ Starts at sleep onset
    - ❑ Reverts on awakening
    - ❑ Idiopathic
    - ❑ Secondary to neurological disorder

MISCELLANEOUS SLEEP DISORDERS EVALUATION AND TREATMENT

1. **INSOMNIA (DIMS=Difficulty initiating and/or maintaining sleep)**
   Insomnia is a common health problem in adults. It affects 10 to 46% of the adult population. It has adverse effects on overall quality of life and economics. Sleep disturbances are associated with increased cardiovascular risk, poor health, depression and decreased quality of life. Sleep complaints are not only a result of aging, but secondary to health burden (medical or psychiatric illnesses, primary sleep disorder or poor sleep hygiene. Most patients do not seek specific treatment. They resign themselves to poor sleep blaming it on stress, aging or illness. Most elderly patients vie insomnia as unavoidable part of the aging process and feel that daytime fatigue is normal. These attitudes constitute barriers to diagnosis of insomnia particularly in the aging population.
   Evaluation:
   - ❑ Patient interview
   - ❑ Bed partner interview
   - ❑ Sleep diaries x 2 weeks
   - ❑ Actigraphy

*ICD-9 codes from the International Classification of Sleep Disorders in parenthesis.

❑ PSG

Differential Diagnosis:
   a. Associated with behavioral/psycho physiological disorders: adjustment sleep disorder, psychophisyological insomnia, inadequate sleep hygiene, limit-setting sleep disorder, sleep-onset association disorder, nocturnal eating (drinking) syndrome and other.
   b. Associated with psychiatric disorders: psychoses, mood disorders, anxiety disorders, panic disorder, alcoholism, other.
   c. Associated with environmental factors: environmental sleep disorder, food allergy insomnia, toxin-induced sleep disorder, other.
   d. Associated with Drug-dependency: Hypnotic, stimulant, alcohol dependent sleep disorder and other.
   e. Associated with sleep-induced respiratory impairment: Obstructive sleep apnea syndrome, central sleep apnea syndrome, central alveolar hypoventilation, COPD, sleep-related asthma, altitude insomnia, other.
   f. Associated with movement disorders: Sleep starts, restless legs syndrome, periodic limb movement disorder, nocturnal leg cramps, rhythmic movement disorder, REM sleep behavior disorder, nocturnal paroxysmal dystonia, other.
   g. Associated with disorders of the timing of the sleep-wake pattern: short sleeper, time zone change (jet lag) syndrome, shift work sleep disorder, delayed sleep phase syndrome, advanced sleep phase syndrome, non-24 hour sleep-wake syndrome, irregular sleep-wake pattern, other.
   h. Associated with parasomnias (not otherwise classified): Confusional arousals, sleep terrors, nightmares, sleep hyperhydrosis, other.
   i. Associated with the Central Nervous System (not otherwise classified): Parkinsonism, Dementia, Cerebral Degenerative Disorders, Sleep Related Epilepsy, Fatal Familial Insomnia, other.
   j. Associated with no objective sleep disturbance: sleep state misperception, sleep choking syndrome, other.
   k. Idiopathic insomnia.
   l. Other: Sleep-related gastro esophageal reflux, fibrositis syndrome, menstrual-associated sleep disorder, pregnancy-associated sleep disorder, terrifying Hypnagogic hallucinations, sleep-related abnormal swallowing syndrome, sleep related laryingospasm, other.

Insomnia treatment:
   ❑ Behavioral treatment primary strategy for:
        o Psycho physiological insomnia
        o Idiopathic insomnia
        o Circadian disorders
        o Inadequate sleep hygiene
   ❑ Behavioral treatment adjunctive strategy for most other chronic insomnias.

*ICD-9 codes from the International Classification of Sleep Disorders in parenthesis.

- Sleep hygiene
- Relaxation techniques
- Stimulus control therapy
  Indications:
  - Psycho physiological insomnia
  - Idiopathic
  - Associated with anxiety disorders
  Instructions to patient:
  - Go to bed only when sleepy
  - If awake for longer than 20-30 minutes, get out of bed, move to a different room, and engage in a monotonous, nonreinforcing activity
  - Return to bed when sleepy
  - Use the bed (bedroom) only for sleep
  - Maintain a regular morning wake-up time
  Goal:
  - Break the conditioned response of "bed and wakefulness"
  - Establish relaxation and sleep as the new conditioned response to BR stimulus.
- Sleep restriction therapy
  Indications:
  - Psycho physiological insomnia
  - Idiopathic
  - Elderly
  - Spends excessive time in bed
  Procedure:
  - Calculate average Total Sleep Time over 2 weeks
  - Establish nightly time in bed = average TST by delaying bed time
  - Keep Wake Time constant
  - Calculate sleep efficiency every 4-5 nights from sleep diary
  - Increase T in Bed by 15 minutes if Sleep efficiency$\geq$ 85% (80% elderly)
  - Frequent follow up
  - Beware of EDS since insomnia pts. Underestimate TST.
  - Results may take 3-5 weeks.
- Cognitive Therapy
  - Maladaptive cognitions:
    - Misattributions of causality
    - Unrealistic expectations for sleep or TX
    - Inaccurate appraisal of consequences of insomnia
  - Educate about sleep and sleep disturbance
  - Suggest more accurate and adaptive thoughts
- Combined behavioral and pharmacologic treatments
  - Long-term benefit of BT may be reduced
  - Effective therapy earlier than BT alone

*ICD-9 codes from the International Classification of Sleep Disorders in parenthesis.

Treatment strategy for Insomnia:
- ❏ Transient or short-term insomnia: treat medical or psychiatric disorder, check for non- prescription medication use. If no response, then use no pharmacological therapies such as stimulus control, sleep restriction, relaxation techniques. If no response, the use short- to intermediate-acting benzodiazepines such as estazolam 0.5mg to 1mg QHS or Zolpidem or Zaleplon (5-20mg QHS). If insufficient response, may use sedating antidepressants such as trazodone (25 to 50mg QHS). And if no response may use combined non-pharmacological and intermittent, sedative-hypnotic when necessary.
- ❏ Chronic insomnia (7-12 weeks or more): start with non-pharmacological therapies with or without sedating antidepressants. If no response, combined treatment.
- ❏ Non-benzodiazepine agents: Imidazopyridines (Zolpidem, alpidem), Pyrazolopyrimidine (Zaleplon), Cyclopyrralone (zopiclone), Sedating antidepressants (trazodone), antihistamines (diphenhydramine), natural remedies (melatonin, valerian).
- ❏ Zolpidem and Zaleplon: Nonbenzodiazepines, act on GABA receptors. They produce less rebound or tolerance and preserve sleep structure. In the elderly they do not increase the risk of falls or respiratory depression and no significant cognitive dysfunction.
- ❏ Over-The-Counter Drugs: Dimenhydrinate (Dramamine) the most frequently used OTD drug by the elderly. Diphenhydramine (Benadryl): may increase AM drowsiness more than prescription hypnotic and may be less efficacious.
- ❏ L-Tryptophan: taken off the market.
- ❏ Melatonin: Increases daytime sleepiness but is it not a good hypnotic. Helps reset the circadian rhythm. It is not FDA regulated so each brand may contain different amounts of Melatonin. May cause headaches and changes in blood pressure. Melatonin sedating effects may be mediated through the GABA system.

SLEEP HYGIENE RECOMMENDATIONS
1. Maintain a regular bedtime and awakening time. Get out of bed at the regular time even if sleep was poor.
2. Do not nap during the day. Regularly scheduled naps if:
   - ❏ Elderly
   - ❏ Shift workers
3. Do not drink alcoholic beverages in the evening.
4. Avoid caffeinated beverages after noontime. Limit total caffeine consumption to no more than two beverages per day.
5. Do not smoke just before bedtime or during the night.
6. Exercise regularly during the day, but avoid exercise in the evening within 3 hours of bedtime
7. Do not use the bed or bedroom for anything other than sleep and sexual activity.

*ICD-9 codes from the International Classification of Sleep Disorders in parenthesis.

8. Establish a relaxing routine in preparation for sleep.
9. Maintain a comfortable temperature in the bedroom.
10. Keep the bedroom dark and quiet.
11. Incorporate social and physical stimulation during the day
12. Increase exposure to bright light during the day.
13. Avoid exposure to bright light during the night.
14. Put aside worries and thoughts about problems
15. Relax, read a book or listen to music before bed.

MEDICATIONS THAT COMMONLY CAUSE INSOMNIA
1. ß-Blockers
2. CST
3. Bronchodilators
4. Respiratory stimulants (theophylline)
5. Stimulating antidepressants
   Protriptyline, fluoxetine, buproprion
6. Methyldopa
7. Thyroid supplements
8. CNS stimulants
9. Decongestants
10. Phenytoin

ERECTILE DISFUNCTION (ED) (780.56-3)
Nocturnal Penile Tumescence (NPT) studies can be performed to differentiate between organic and psychological causes of impotence. Normally during REM sleep there are spontaneous non-sexual related penile erections. An increase of 2 cm in penile circumference indicates an erection. The average penile circumference is 8 cm. An 18 year old spends 200 minutes of TST with an erection, this time decreases after 30 years of age and by 40 year is usually 100 minutes of sleep time. The amount of pressure generated by the erect penis is 1 kg in the normal subject. The minimal amount necessary to penetrate is 500 grams.
In a NTP study, the measures taken are:
1. The Tmax which is the time maintaining an erection, usually 40 % of REM sleep.
2. Tup is measured from the beginning of an erection to the Tmax and
3. Tdown from the beginning of the detumescence to Tzero, where there is no erection any more.

Risk Factors for Erectile Dysfunction (ED)

- Diabetes
- Arteriosclerosis
- Peripheral Vascular Disease
- Cardiovascular Disease
- Hypertension
- Renal Failure and Dialysis

*ICD-9 codes from the International Classification of Sleep Disorders in parenthesis.

- Pelvic Injury or Surgery
- Spinal Cord Injury
- Neurologic Conditions
- Endocrine Abnormalities
- Lipoprotein Abnormalities
- Anger, Anxiety or Depression
- Cigarette Smoking
- Drug Abusers
- Alcohol and Alcoholism
- Sleep Disordered Breathing

Causes of iatrogenic ED:
- Sympatholytics: they prolong detumescence
- Antidepressants, except imipramine that inhibits REM, but not tumescence. The less likely to affect NPT are Trimipramine and buproprion (no REM effect), Nefazodone (serzone) Increase REM and NPT slightly, but no rebound.
- Antiandrogenics
- Antipsychotics
- Tagamet
- Disulfiram
- Atropine
- Digoxin
- Cancer chemotherapeutics

Treatment depends on cause. May use vacuum pump with band, injection therapy, drugs such as Sildefanil (Viagra). Urologic referral is recommended.

ENURESIS (780.56-0)

*ICD-9 codes from the International Classification of Sleep Disorders in parenthesis.

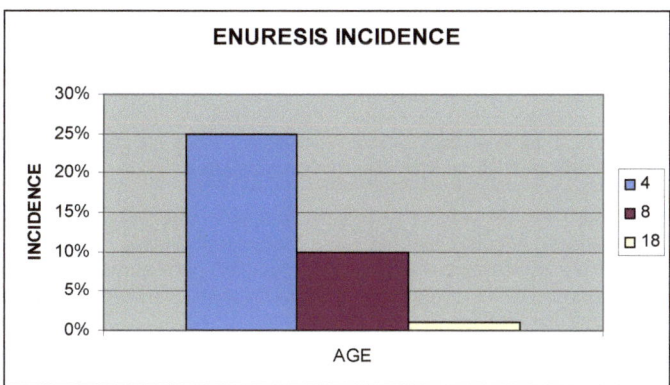

The incidence of enuresis decreases with age as seen on the above graph. By the age of 4, 25% of children have enuresis, 10% of the eight year olds and 1% of 18 year olds. Secondary enuresis has a third of the incidence of primary enuresis. The incidence of spontaneous resolution is 12-15% per year. If the patient is more than 6 years old, a work up is necessary to exclude other problems such as:
  a) Urologic: Acquired (UTI) or congenital.
  b) Constipation
  c) Diabetes Mellitus
  d) Cerebral Palsy
  e) OSA

Treatment of Enuresis: Imipramine (has equal success than conditioning training), DDAVP and Behavioral Therapy (waking child at regular intervals, rewards, keeping a diary).

KLEIN-LEVINE SYNDROME (780.54-2) Cyclical periodic hyper somnolence and hyper sexuality occurring most frequently in adolescent boys. They have sleep onset REM sleep (SOREM) and decreased slow wave sleep (SWS). The differential diagnosis is with Narcolepsy and Depression.

CONFUSIONAL AROUSALS (307.46-2)
Confusional arousals are partial arousals that occur from Slow Wave Sleep. The patient appears confused upon awakening from sleep. They can be induced by forced arousal. There is absence of fear, walking or intense hallucinations. They are not associated with seizure activity on EEG.

SLEEP TERRORS (307.46-1)

*ICD-9 codes from the International Classification of Sleep Disorders in parenthesis.

Prevalence: 6% of children, with a peak incidence at 5 to 7 years of age and another peak during adolescence. The most important factor is genetic predisposition. The triggers for sleep walking (SW) and sleep terrors (ST) are the same: sleep deprivation, fever, stress, drugs, and sensory (auditory) stimuli during sleep.

All arousal disorders arise in NREM sleep. There is amnesia of event. For sleep walking the best strategy is to gently guide the sleepwalker to a sleeping place.

The treatment for ST and SW is the same. Reassurance, as these conditions tend to decrease with age. May use benzodiazepine, hypnotics if necessary. Formal evaluation is required if disruptive or violent behavior occurs to rule out other parasomnias such as Unusual nocturnal seizures, RBD, Psychogenic or other dissociative conditions such as fugue and multiple personality disorder.

NIGHT SWEATS (SLEEP HYPERHIDROSIS) (780.8)
There is an increase of sweating at the beginning of SWS and a decrease during REM. The differential diagnosis is:
1. Diabetes Insipidus
2. Hypotension
3. Hyperthyroidism
4. Hypoglycemia
5. Hot Flashes
6. Infection
7. Chronic Fatigue syndrome
8. Hodgkin's Disease
9. OSA (65% incidence, occurs due to intermittent sympathomimetic discharges during hypoxemic state)
10. GERD
11. Pheocromocitoma
12. Hypothalamic lesions
13. Epilepsy
14. Stroke
15. Cerebral Palsy
16. Chronic paroxysmal hemi crania
17. Spinal Cord Infarction
18. Head Injury
19. Typhus
20. Brucellosis
21. Plague
22. Familial Dysautonomia
23. Pregnancy
24. Antipyretics

EXCESSIVE DAYTIME SLEEPINESS (EDS)
Differential Diagnosis:

*ICD-9 codes from the International Classification of Sleep Disorders in parenthesis.

About 5% of the population complains of being sleepy during the day, however this symptom is subjective.
1. Sleep disordered breathing: OSA, Upper Airway Resistance Syndrome. OSA is the most common cause seen in medical practice.
2. Drug use: antihistaminic, tranquilizing.
3. Withdrawal from stimulants: coffee, cocaine, OTC stimulants.
4. Circadian Rhythm Disorders: Jet Lag and shift work.
5. PLM, other parasomnias
6. CNS problems: Idiopathic Hypersomnia and Narcolepsy (EDS presents during the second decade of life).
7. Infections: EBV, ECHO, Hepatitis virus.
8. After bout of Infectious Mononucleosis, Atypical pneumonia, Hepatitis, aseptic meningitis or during the course of encephalitis or hydrocephalus.
9. Idiopathic
10. Poor sleep hygiene

UPPER AIRWAY RESISTANCE SYNDROME
1. Progressive increase in respiratory efforts. Excessive negative esophageal pressure with nadirs between -13 to -51 cmH2O (Normal is more or equal to -8) also there is decreased Peak Flow and Tidal Volume 1-2 breaths before arousal.
2. Snoring
3. Arousals. No Desaturation no hyponeas or apneas.
4. Decreased sleep latency in MSLT.
5. Complains of excessive daytime sleepiness due to disrupted sleep.

THERAPY FOR SLEEP DISORDERED BREATHING
1. **SNORING:** Dependent on the problem UPPP, Nasal septoplasty, nasal steroids, nasal chromolyn, and oral appliances are available, as well as ear plugs for the patient and his/her bed partner, since snoring may lead to deafness.
2. **SURGERY FOR OSA:** Tracheostomy, only one curative in 100% of patients. Pharyngoplasty, nasal and genioplasty, depending on the problem at hand.
3. **O2:** eliminates PVC's, ST-Tw changes, transient PHTN. Improves "hypoxic EEG (SW)", increases sleep quality, and prolongs life only if given at least for 18 hours in patients with severe COPD. It does not cause brady-tachy arrhythmias. Does not require sleep study unless insurance requires approval for resting wake SPO2 more than 55.
4. **Progesterone:** Increases the Tidal Volume.
5. **CPAP:** useful to treat Central apneas, but it may also cause central apneas perhaps due to hypocapnia or lung distension. In pure central Apneas CPAP is corrective. It corrects hypoxemia, decreases CO2 stores and increases EF in CHF. CPAP= Increases FRC, decreases work of breathing (WOB) and splints the airway.

*ICD-9 codes from the International Classification of Sleep Disorders in parenthesis.

6. **BIPAP:** is like Pressure Support with PEEP on the ventilator. It is initiated by the patient's flow trigger, hence do not use in patients with decreased ventilatory drive unless a rate is used as well (S/T mode). Also splints the airway, increases the FRC and decreases the WOB and pCO2. Most helpful in pts with high pCO2. The driving pressure is the IPAP-EPAP gradient.

7. **CPAP COMPLIANCE:** 5 hours/day and 91% of the time at its effective pressure. Follow up is important to increase compliance.
   BiPAP does not improve compliance. Heated humidifiers do.

8. Split night studies decrease compliance. The final pressure in later half of night may not be sufficient and may require the patient to come back at another night for more titration.

9. **AutoCPAP: Auto CPAP** is a CPAP unit that through a proprietary method depending on the manufacturer has a mechanism by which the machine senses airway resistance and delivers the amount of pressure required to maintain the airway open. So if during NREM sleep the patient does not have apneas the machine will deliver the lowest limit of pressure allowed. If the patient starts having events because REM sleep started, then the machine will sense the resistance and deliver the pressure required. If the patient is awake or snoring, also the machine will deliver the pressure required to overcome snoring or the lowest if the airway is open as when the patient is awake.
   For unselected patients, AutoCPAP has not been proved to substantially increase adherence, but those patients that do not tolerate CPAP may accept auto CPAP better. AutoCPAP may help in postural OSA where there are large variations in pressure requirements, REM associated OSA, pressure sensitive patients, patients with high mouth leak on higher pressure or patients on high pressures.
   AutoCPAP has not been recommended for unattended Auto CPAP titration for routine practice. May use in hospitalized patients with partially attended titration in telemetry with oximetry and respiratory therapist to adjust a leak or in the ICU with oxymetry, EKG and respiratory therapist as well.

10. **Cheine-Stokes Breathing (CSB):** Temazepam is safe to control arousals induced by CSB, but CSB continues. Nasal CPAP leads to the feeling of not enough air during the hyperpneic phase, BiPAP may work better, but O2 is the best.

UNIHEMISPHERIC SLEEP
Dolphins, porpoises and whales have unihemispheric sleep. The first two lack REM sleep.

SLEEP REGULATION
Suprachiasmatic Nucleus: Circadian rhythm pacemaker.
Ultradian rhythm: less than 24 hours
Infradian rhythm: more than 24 hours
Circannual rhythm: periods on the order of a year.

Growth Hormone (GH): GH secretion has multiple peaks in females in all stages of sleep, day and night. In males GH peaks during stages 3 and 4 only.

*ICD-9 codes from the International Classification of Sleep Disorders in parenthesis.

Prolactin: Prolactin levels increase with sleep. Hyperprolactinemia does not produce sleepiness.

Cortisol: This hormone has a sleep related cycle, similar to the temperature cycle. Cortisol levels remain the same during the lifetime of an individual, unlike others hormones levels that become flatter with age. ACTH and Cortisol levels are reduced during REM sleep. In major depression, Cortisol levels are elevated all day.

TSH: non-sleep cycle. One hour after sleep onset there is a sharp decrease in TSH, consistent with the decrease in body temperature.

LH: There is a surge of LH between the hours of 3 and 10 AM, not related with sleep but with time of the day.

Melatonin: Only secreted in dark. Blind people have a free running melatonin secretion. Lowers body temperature by half in humans. The physiologic level is 0.1 to 0.3. A dose of 0.1mg of Melatonin halves the sleep latency from the normal of 15-20' to 7.5 minutes. Pharmacologic levels are in the range of 1 to 3 mg, and at doses of 1 gram Melatonin has soporific effects.

Tryptophan: Tryptophan is an essential amino acid and precursor of Serotonin and Serotonin is a precursor of Melatonin, hence Tryptophan has soporiphic effects. Tryptophan was taken off the market.

Hypothyroidism: Severe hypothyroidism leads to lethargy and increased Total Sleep Time. Mixedema increases the risk of OSA due to mixedema of the upper airway, but OSA is not correlated with hypothyroidism.

Neglect: Neglect in children leads to failure to thrive and decreased levels of Growth hormone and Slow Wave Sleep (SWS) that return to normal levels when nurturing the child.

Circadian rhythm and sleep: The free running circadian rhythm is about 25 hours, so every morning our clock has to adjust 1 hour backwards. Hence it is easier to adjust to a shift in sleep forward and to westbound travel. When crossing time zones towards the west, time is hours ahead of the zone of origin. The ability to adjust to the difference in our internal clock and the 24-hour day imposed by society is decreased as we age, particularly after the age of 35. We synchronize our circadian rhythm in the morning. Phase is a point in a rhythm. Exercise and/or light in the morning phase advance the sleep cycle and if exercise or light exposure occurs in the evening, there will be a phase delay. In other words, exercising in the morning will tend to make us sleepy earlier at night. If we exercise in the evening we will be sleepy late at night.

*ICD-9 codes from the International Classification of Sleep Disorders in parenthesis.

During travel the circadian rhythm adjusts at 1.5h/d going west and 1h/d going east. One day per Time Zone crossed is required for adaptation. The maximum tendency to fall asleep occurs between 4:00-5:00 hours and 15:30 to 16:30 hours. The peak of alertness is at 9:30 AM after a night of sleep and between 19:30 to 21:30 hours. The Body temperature through occurs around 3:00 hours, at this time Cortisol levels start raising and peak at about 07:00 hours. The body temperature first peak is at around 7:00 PM and it starts declining steadily after that time. In the advanced phase sleep disorder both body temperature and body Cortisol rhythms are advanced as well.

CHEMICALS AND SLEEP
1. **WAKING:** Regular and tonic discharge of neurons.
   - Catecholamines (DA, NE, Epi)
   - Acetylcholine (lower dose than in REM)
   - Histamine
   - Glutamate
   - CSF-borne factors & peptides: Wake-promoting factor, substance P, CRF & TRF, VIP
   - Blood borne factors: Epinephrine,
   - Histamine, Glucocorticosteroids.
2. **REM:** Burst-pause discharge of neurons. Ventral to locus ceruleans. Critical for REM. NE synthesis is decreased during REM. Acetylcholine (Ach) stimulates REM sleep.
3. **SWS:** low levels of Ach
   - Serotonin
   - Adenosine+ Caffeine
   - GABA
   - CSF-peptides
   - Opiate peptides: Encephalin, endorphins.
   - Somatostatin
   - PGD2
   - Uridine
   - Blood: Serotonin, Insulin Cholecystokinin, bombesin, Muramyl peptide, IL-1, delta sleep inducing peptide
   - **Neuroleptics:** Inhibit DA, H1 and α receptors. AntiDopaminergics.

SLEEP ONTOGENY
Infants at birth sleep 17 to 18 hours per day. Fifty percent of sleep time is active sleep. There are 3-5 episodes of sleep distributed over the day and night equally. At the beginning, sleep has an active onset. Years later NREM sleep onset develops.

At three months, the baby starts sleeping more during the night. At four months, the four stages of NREM appear on the sleep EEG. By 4-5 years of age, the sleep period is monophasic, i.e.: sleep occurs once every 24 hours.

*ICD-9 codes from the International Classification of Sleep Disorders in parenthesis.

Overtime, there is a decrease in total sleep time (TST) and in REM %. By 4 years of age, the TST is about 10-12 hours. By 10 years of age, TST is about 9-10 hours. During adolescence, TST is 7-9 hours.

REM% during childhood is about 25-35%, by puberty it becomes 20% of TST.

NEWBORN EEG (*conceptual age=CA)
Trace discontinue: Long periods of quiescence awake and sleep since birth.

Sleep Ontogeny:
At CA of 30 wks- REM continuous activity
At CA or 34 wks- REM and wake continuous
At 32 NREM starts. AT 37-38 wks NREM is continuous. From 38 wks CA to 5 wks post term trace alternant (decrease voltage) during NREM.
At less than 6 months, sleep consists of active, quiet and indeterminate periods.
At more than 6 months he infant's sleep stages are the same than in adults.

Beta-delta complexes: during the first 26 wks of conceptual age.

Theta burst: "saw tooth waves". First at 26 wks CA. At 33 wks alpha burst are more prominent.
Frontal sharp waves: At 34 wks CA. Vertex sharp waves not seen in REM.

Difference in sleep and waking EEG: not until 36-37 wks CA. Beta-delta complexes until 37 wks CA. After 36 wks CA until the second month post-term there are changes in wake EEG. The background is low voltage random semirhytmic 4-8 Hz. Disappearance of Beta-delta complexes in awake.

Alpha rhythm: rare in neonates. Seen in chromosomal abnormalities or inborn errors of metabolism. It occurs in 75% of normal babies more than 3-4 month old.

Hypsarrhythmia: Abnormal pattern. Burst of high voltage and spikes diffusely asynchronous. At 44 wks or later CA presents in its classical pattern. Less than 44 wks it presents as variant suppression-burst pattern. Burst duration is one second or more, the amplitude is up to 1000mV (other patterns have an amplitude of 250 mV or less). Spasms may occur during attenuation periods. In neonates it is called "early infantile epileptic encephalopathy" secondary to brain malfunction. "Neonatal myoclonic encephalopathy" begins in the first few wks of life with myoclonus, seizures and suppression-burst EEG secondary to brain malfunction and inborn errors of metabolism.

NORMAL SLEEP EEG

*ICD-9 codes from the International Classification of Sleep Disorders in parenthesis.

Children demonstrate increased wave amplitude and with age amplitude decreases. Therefore, in elderly patients we may need to increase the sensitivity of the EEG (10mm=25mV) and in children we need to decrease the sensitivity (10mm=100 mV).

The Low Frequency Filter is decreased to eliminate slow artifacts and the High Frequency Filter is decreased to eliminate fast artifacts.

To increase the amplitude of brain waves, distance between electrodes is maximized. Reference C3 to A2 and C4 to A1.

> **Occipital alpha waves (Occ α):** occur during relaxation with eyes closed. By 3 years of age they have a frequency of 8 Hertz (Hz=cycles per second or CPS). Their frequency increases with age and in adults the frequency range is between 8 to 13 Hz with an average of 10 Hz.
>
> Factors that slow the frequency of alpha waves are: brain hypo perfusion, Carbamazepine in children even at therapeutic levels and Dilantin only at toxic levels.
>
> A Permanent Pacemaker increases the alpha rate by about 2 Hz.
>
> **Alpha wave frequency ontogeny:** 75% of normal babies between 3-4 months after term births have occipital rhythm activity that resolves upon eye opening. The initial alpha frequency is 3.5 to 4.5 Hz. The mean alpha frequency by 12 months reaches 5-6 Hz in 70% of babies. By 36 months 8 Hz in 82%, by 9 years of age, 9 Hz in 65% of children and by 15 years of age, 10 Hz in 65% of children. In the elderly there is a decline in alpha frequency by 58 years of age with a mean of 9 Hz.
>
> Eye opening may totally block alpha frequency in infants and young children. In adults there is an attenuation of alpha waves.
>
> **Voltage:** the longer the distance between electrodes, the higher the amplitude of EEG waves, however geometry and potential field also determine EEG wave amplitude. EEG wave amplitude decreases with increasing age due to changes in bone density and increase electrode impedance of intervening tissues. EEG's done with electrodes directly on brain tissue do not show a decrease in impedance with aging.
>
> **Distribution of alpha rhythm:** There are multiple generators. There is overlap and influence between each generator. 65% of adults and 95% of children have maximum alpha voltage in the occipital lobe. 32% of normal young adolescent have wide distribution or predominately central or temporal or equal distribution of alpha rhythm.

*ICD-9 codes from the International Classification of Sleep Disorders in parenthesis.

Bilateral Symmetry: The occipital alpha rhythm is asymmetric in 60% of adults: The differences are 50% higher amplitude in the right hemisphere, regardless of handedness and less than 20% difference between right and left. In 1.5% of adults there is a difference between right and left greater than 50%. If more than 30-50% difference in amplitude exists, were the left is higher than the right, a structural lesion such as scalp swelling secondary to hematoma from leaking injured scalp veins, may be present.

Mu rhythm: This rhythm is central, 8-10 Hz. 19% of adults have, the gender difference is 2:1, female: male. It is blocked with contra lateral movement of extremities. It is related inversely to the level of attention, the higher the attention the more suppressed the Mu rhythm is. It is increased by immobility. The voltage increases by absence of bone (burr hole) and may be unilateral.

Beta activity: Also central. More than 12 Hz. The amplitude is less or equal to 25 mV. Beta activity presents in three bands, the most common is 18-25 Hz, also seen in Stages I, II and REM. The 14-16 Hz band is less common and the 3-40 Hz is rare and seen in psychosis. The amplitude increases with drugs such as barbiturates and continues in the wake state. If there is a focal decrease in amplitude more or equal to 50% it is abnormal, it represents cortical depression due to ischemia, atrophy, cystic deficiency, intervening fluid (scalp edema, epidural bleed).
Generalized increased voltage with anterior dominance indicates brain damage. Continuous spindling and fast activity during sleep is seen in mental retardation and cerebral palsy.

Theta activity: Also central, 6-7 Hz, voltage less or equal to 15 mV. Increases as alpha rhythm disappears with drowsiness.
Beta waves: more than 13 cps, less than 25mV: Stages I, II, REM

Alpha waves (α): 8-13 cps (cycles per second)

Delta waves: 1-3 cps, more than 75 mV

Theta waves (Θ): 4-7 cps, less than 15 mV, REM and Stage II

Spindle: 12-18cps
V waves: over center or vertex of scalp, 200 mV negative (upward) deflection followed by shorter positive deflection (downward), in stage I or 2, not in deep sleep.
Frequency: Spindle >α(alpha) >Θ(theta) >delta

CPS: 12-18>8-13>3-7>1-2
Mnemonic: S>A>T>D "SeATeD"
Slow wave amplitude: less age=greater amplitude, hence, in a 15 year old, the delta amplitude is in the 100 mV range, while in the elderly it is 75 mV. This

*ICD-9 codes from the International Classification of Sleep Disorders in parenthesis.

may be due to decreased skull bone density, since electrodes placed directly on brain reveal no difference in delta wave amplitude with aging.

Definitions:

Sleep Onset: Lights Out to first set of 3 consecutive epochs of Stage 1 or first epoch of any other stage.

Stage I: Monorhythmic, slow. Slow pendular eye movements, disappearance of occipital alpha rhythm, appearance of rhythmic fronto-central and central theta activity. Four to six Hz indicates drowsiness in infants more than 3 months of age and children less than 9 years old. Bursts of high voltage more than 350 mV slow wave that disappears in deeper sleep.

Arousal: Initially dysphasic slow wave, vertex sharp wave (erroneously called "K complex") followed by rapid oscillations 8-14 Hz, and/or evidence of further arousal (change in sleep stage). Before 2 months of age neither component of arousal occurs. Only transient Desynchronization. At 8-12 weeks, there is a rudimentary slow wave response to stimuli. By 3 months there is a well-defined slow wave component. The faster component can be seen by 7 months of age, initially rudimentary few moderate high voltage sinusoidal waves 4-4.5 Hz that with increasing age achieve the 8-10 Hz seen in adult. Arousals last 4-5 seconds, rarely more than 30 seconds.
Arousals in adults: From Stage I, reverse to wake alpha rhythm. From Stage II and above, more attenuated form than the one seen in children. Initially dysphasic central, followed by brief alpha wave in fronto-central area.

SENSORY THRESHOLD FOR AROUSAL.
The sensory threshold for arousal is greater in REM than in NREM in animals and humans. Among the NREM stages, the deeper the stage, the higher the threshold. The younger the subject the higher the threshold as well.

Hence with increasing age, the auditory threshold for arousal decreases. By 62 years of age, the sensory threshold for arousal is 60 decibels (DBLS), which occurs, in normal conversation. By 44 years of age, 70 decibels or the sound produced by a car. By 22 years of age, 80 DBLS or the noise produced by a bus. In childhood the sensory threshold is 123 decibels or the noise produced by a rock concert.

Flurazepam increases the sensory threshold for arousal by 5 to 30 decibels. A smoke alarm produces 85 decibels, so the question is raised whether a fire alarm will awake a person taking sedatives or that is sleep deprived.

Insomniacs report them selves as "light sleepers"; however their auditory arousal threshold is not different than in normal subjects.

*ICD-9 codes from the International Classification of Sleep Disorders in parenthesis.

EEG ACTIVITY OF SLEEP

Vertex Sharp wave Transients: Stages II and IV. They Signal the onset of Stage II. Maximum voltage seen in C3 and C4. Usually diphasic, negative deflection (up) followed by a low voltage positive deflection down. May be followed by a slow negative wave or spindle. They appear for the first time at 8 weeks of age. Always symmetrical. Asymmetry indicates a lesion such as hydrocephalus. They may occur in quick succession (every 1-2 seconds) in an interference pattern.

K complexes and vertex transients: 0.5-2 Hz
They occur in response to auditory stimuli. They are similar to vertex sharp waves in amplitude, voltage, configuration and frequency. Does not occur spontaneous only secondary to stimuli and they have about 5 minute refractory period and may disappear if stimuli is repeated over 30" or more. They occur in Stages II, III and rarely in IV.

Spindles: Fronto-central. Average frequency of 14 Hz, range 12-16 Hz. Duration: 0.5-1.5", several seconds in children. Spindles appear for the first time by 6-8 weeks of age. At that time they are bilateral and asynchronous. Synchronization increases during the first year of life up to 18 month when they are most synchronous. In infants they last 2-4", not fusiform, sharply peaked in surface negative phase, similar to Mu rhythm. There are three types of spindles:
1. 14 Hz/C3, C4: In adults, occur in stages 2, 3 and in sleep coma.
2. 10-12 Hz/Frontal: 5% of 3-12 year olds. Less than 3-second duration.
3. 10 Hz continuous: cerebral palsy, mentally retarded children, drugs such as morphine and halothane. Need to differentiate with sigma rhythm, which is 18-22 Hz, fusiform unremitting burst in sleep that do not occur in response to stimuli and are secondary to phenothiazines, barbiturates or in children in pathologic conditions.

Fast Activity: Rare after 7 years of age. Starts at 5-6 months. Low voltage fast at sleep onset, 28 Hz +/- 6 Hz. Low amplitude less or equal to 5 mV, 30 mV at 12-18 mo, at 30-36 months, the amplitude decreases and it becomes less pronounced.

Sedation: Increases fast activity in awake and sleep. Maximum voltage in stages II and III. Upon arousal the fast activity becomes more pronounced than before sleep unless chronic medication use were during pre and post arousal the fast activity does not change. More than 30% asymmetry indicates a low side lesion.

Positive occipital Sharp Transient (POST of sleep): Sharp positive deflection followed by low voltage negative deflection. It looks like a check mark. May be about 60% asymmetric.

Occipital Slow Transients: In children from light sleep to deep sleep, bilateral high voltage occipital slow transients. Cone shaped to diphasic similar to slow vertex

*ICD-9 codes from the International Classification of Sleep Disorders in parenthesis.

transient. At first equal than 3-6 second with deeper sleep, more frequent and melt with delta waves. They may be negative or biphasic negative-positive.

SLEEP POLYSOMNOGRAPHY (PSG)

C4-A1, O1-A2 (alpha activity), T3-Cz and Cz-T4 (spindles and V waves).

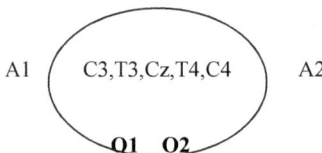

A1   C3,T3,Cz,T4,C4   A2

O1   O2

Electrode placement Diagram.

Electrodes are placed and referenced bilaterally in case one gets disrupted to be able to use another electrode without waking the patient up.

The paper speed in routine EEG is 30mm/", in the sleep EEG is 10-15mm/". Filter settings are: Low frequency filter (LFF) 0.3Hz and 35 Hz for the High frequency filter (HFF). For EMG the LFF is 10 Hz and the HFF at 70Hz.

The amplifier sensitivity is set at 50-100 mV/10mm. The most used is 70mV/10mm.

During REM the rapid slope is less than 300mseconds and amplitude more than 200 mV. When the pupil moves to the electrode it produces a positive (down) deflection and when it moves away there is a negative deflection (up) in the EEG. Since eyes movements are conjugate, the deflection for the right eye will be opposite direction than the one on the left eye channel.

The chin EMG identifies REM and movement arousal. The sensitivity is set at 2 mV/mm.

Paradoxical breathing: occurs when there is an increase in the thoracic circumpherence with a decrease in abdominal circumpherence, it is commonly seen in OSA.

One Epoch =1 page, 10mm/"=30"

SUMMARY OF SLEEP PSG SCORING

Wake: alpha activity or low voltage/mixed frequency activity, REM's, Blinks and tonic EMG activity.

*ICD-9 codes from the International Classification of Sleep Disorders in parenthesis.

REM = Low Voltage/mixed frequency activity. Episodic REM's. Saw-tooth waves (2-5 Hz) vertex negative waves before rapid eye movements (REM's). There is lack of tone in EMG, no K complexes and no spindles. Three minute rule: No REM's between K complexes or spindles, revert scoring to stage II.

Stage I: More than 50% of the epoch has low voltage 2-7 Hz frequency. V waves occur late. Slow rolling eye movements, absent K complexes and absent spindles. Tonic EMG activity less than wake.

Stage II: Spindles or K complexes occur in stages II through IV. Less than 20% delta. Spindles last more than 0.5". K complexes last more than 0.5" and are biphasic vertex waves. The 3' rule= more than 3' between spindles or K complexes=stage I (SI) or wake. Arousal between 3' the next stage would be stage I or wake.

Stage III: 20-50% delta: 2Hz and more than 75mV-SWS.

Stage IV: More than 50% delta, it is the actual time of delta waves.

Movement Time: when more than 50% of the epoch is obscured by movement artifact.

Awakening: return to awake sustained more than 30". Must include an increase in EMG tone in REM sleep, not in NREM sleep.

Arousal: At least 10" of sleep between arousals. Abrupt change in EEG frequency.

1. Return of alpha activity less than 30 ".
2. Low voltage fast activity
3. Rhythmic slow wave activity more than 2-4 "
4. Shift to a lighter sleep stage and increase in EMG activity, also more than 2-4 ".
5. Series (more than 3 or 4) V waves and increase in EMG activity, more than 2-4".

PLM's: 0.5-4" duration every 5"-120" (4 epochs) and equal or more than 5 movements in a cluster.

Movement Associated Arousal: Arousal occurring 2-4" before or after a PLM in the absence of other event.

Movement Index: PMS/hour of sleep.

Movement-Arousal Index (MAI): #PMS+Arousals/hour. This index is better correlated to sleep disruption than the movement index.

Sleep Onset Latency: In the MSLT, sleep onset is defined as the time from lights out (LO) to the first epoch of any stage of sleep. In the PSG, sleep onset latency is the time from LO to the third epoch of stage I, or the first epoch of any other stage. Normal at night is 15-20', during MSLT more than 10 minutes.

REM Latency: Time from Lights Out to REM minus epochs of awakenings. Normal 70-120'.

Total Recording Time: Wake+NREM+REM+Movement time

Total Sleep Time: NREM+REM

Sleep Efficiency: Total Sleep Time/Total Recording Time*100.

REM Sleep latency: Time from sleep onset to first epoch of stage REM.

*ICD-9 codes from the International Classification of Sleep Disorders in parenthesis.

Atypical Sleep Patterns:

1. *Alpha-Delta Sleep:* 5-20% delta waves plus alpha rhythm with high amplitude at 7-10 Hz.
2. *REM spindle:* 1-8% of sleep in normal subjects, also in narcoleptics and hypersominacs.
3. *SOREM:* REM within 15 minutes of sleep onset. It is seen in narcoleptics, sleep deprivation, irregular sleep-wake habits, ETOH or drug withdrawal, severe depression and as a marker of endogenous depression.
4. *REM without atonia:* It is seen in RBD, tricyclic antidepressants and untreated narcolepsy.

Awakening in MSLT: 2 epochs of wake after sleep onset.

Narcolepsy:

      1) 2 REM onset naps + mean Sleep Latency less or equal to 5-8 minutes.
      2) Cataplexy

If only 1 SOREM, repeat MSLT. If SO is less or equal to 5 minutes and there are no SOREM's then consider CNS Hypersomnia.
If the MSLT SO is between 5-10 minutes, repeat and if the repeat study is normal, and then may rule out episodic hypersomnia such as menstrual hypersomnia syndrome or Klein-Levin Syndrome.

REM: Any section contiguous with REM is REM if it has low voltage plus mixed frequency plus decreased EMG tone, with or without rapid eye movement, in the absence of arousals.
However, a segment between two spindles without REM's more than 15" is scored as stage 2.

Obstructive Apnea: if Central apnea less than 25% of total apnea.

Mixed Apnea: if central component predominates 25-90% of event.

Central apnea: 90-100% is central apnea.

Arousals:
    1. Chin EMG increase without EEG changes.
    2. Changes in sleep stage or alpha less than 15".
    3. Alpha rhythm more than 15".

PSG PEARLS

*ICD-9 codes from the International Classification of Sleep Disorders in parenthesis.

CYCLICAL VARIATION OF THE HEART RATE (CVHR)

- ❏ Absolute change in HR of 9 or more BPM with subsequent return to baseline
- ❏ Cycle lengths 15-45 "
- ❏ Minimum 3 consecutive cycles
- ❏ More than 20-50% of each epoch has CVHR
- ❏ CVHR has positive correlation with OSA:
  - ○ If 20% of each epoch and less than 5% of all epochs have CVHR:
    - 95% sensitivity for OSA
    - 28% specificity
    - 88% negative PV
  - ○ If 50% of each epoch and more 15% of all epochs have CVHR:
    - 98% specificity
    - 95% positive PV
    - 47% sensitivity

AROUSALS

- ❏ Increased EEG frequency or EMG artifact in EEG more than 20"plus increased EMG amplitude

OSA ARRYTHMIAS

- ❏ Sinus Arrest: Pauses greater than 2.5" : 10 % incidence in OSA
- ❏ 5% 2nd. AV Block.
- ❏ 3% Ventricular Tachycardia.
- ❏ 20% PVC's. (Correlates with severity of decrease in SpO2 < 60%)
- ❏ The majority of arrhythmias are unrelated to OSA, some may resolve with O2.
- ❏ Evaluation: History and Physical Exam plus ECG to rule out structural Heart Disease.   Individualize therapy according to risk of CVS morbi-mortality.

GERD

- ❏ Distal esophageal pH less than 4 during more than 30".
- ❏ Normal distal esophageal pH= 5.5-6.5. Sleep increases clearance time.
- ❏ Reflux rare after 2 h postprandial in normal supine patients.
- ❏ Increased REM in Irritable Bowel Syndrome.
- ❏ **Rx:**
  - **a.** Elevate the head of the bed
  - **b.** Bethanecol: decreases the frequency of episodes by 35% Decreases Clearance by 53%,
  - **c.** Increases Peristalsis and Lower Esophageal Sphincter tone.
  - **d.** H2 blockers: BID for GERD due to postprandial reflux unlike duodenal ulcer.
      Pepcid 40 mg qhs
      20mg or 40 mg BID
  - **e.** CPAP: Decreases GERD in pts with and without OSA.

*ICD-9 codes from the International Classification of Sleep Disorders in parenthesis.

f. Discontinue ETOH 3 or more hours before bedtime. ETOH increases Clearance time.

g. Discontinue Benzodiazepines (They increase Clearance time and decrease arousal index).

DECREASED REM LATENCY: REM Latency is the interval between Stage 1 and REM. This interval does not change with normal aging.

- Infancy
- Depression and other mood Disorders: excess Acetylcholine, Increased sensitivity to cholinergic REM sleep induction (decreased REM latency), increased REM % and time, increased density of rapid eye movements and there is flattening of REM periods, i.e.: no change in the duration of REM periods across the night (normal: progressive prolongation of REM periods). Increased nocturnal temperature and flattening of temperature curve and circadian rhythm. Decreased SWS, decreased delta sleep inducing CSF peptide in Depression and Schizophrenia. REM deprivation is effective in depressed mood disorders but not in Schizophrenia. This maneuver may trigger mania. In depression there is also an increase in Sleep Latency. There is a decrease in sleep associated Growth Hormone secretion. Upon early relapse of Depression, there is decreased REM latency and decreased delta sleep.
- Schizophrenia: decreased S4 sleep.
- ETOH abuse
- Borderline Personality Disorder.
- Narcolepsy
- Eating Disorder
- Panic Disorder
- PTSD
- Schizoaffective Disorder.
- Withdrawal from TCA's, Benzodiazepines , ETOH
- Recovery from sleep deprivation
- Shift work
- Jet Lag
- Circadian Rhythm disorder

REM sleep is associated with increased Acetylcholine and decreased Serotonin and NE.

MULTIPLE SLEEP LATENCY TEST (MSLT)

The MSLT is a tool used to assess the degree of a patient's sleepiness and also a tool to support the diagnosis of Narcolepsy. The MSLT is conducted with the patient dressed in street clothes after a full night of polysomnography testing. Two hours after the PSG is finished, a series of at least four (five are required for the diagnosis of narcolepsy) 20 minutes naps at 2-hour intervals are conducted. Averages for sleep latency across the four naps of less than 5 minutes are considered pathological, the normal is 10-20 minutes, and 5-10 is a gray area. Two or more sleep-onset REM episodes are diagnostic of narcolepsy, and it is found in 80% of patient with this condition. In sleep-deprived patients, such as those with sleep-disordered breathing, this assumption should be made after the

*ICD-9 codes from the International Classification of Sleep Disorders in parenthesis.

underlying condition such as sleep apnea has been treated and normalization of nocturnal sleep proved upon reevaluation.

Mild Sleepiness is defined as sleep episodes that occur during times of rest or where little attention is required and is usually associated with a MSLT mean sleep latency of 10-15 minutes. It is found in normal subjects.

Moderate sleepiness is defined as episodes of sleep that are present daily during very mild physical activities requiring at most a moderate degree of alertness such as driving, attending movies, or similar group meetings. It produces moderate impairment in social or occupational function. The MSLT mean sleep latency is in the gray zone between 5 and 10 minutes.

Severe sleepiness is defined as sleep episodes present daily at times of physical activity requiring mild to moderate attention such as eating, conversation, driving, walking. The social or occupational function is markedly impaired. The mean MSLT sleep latency is less than 5 minutes and the patient should be warned about a potential industrial or motor vehicle accident.

Toxicology screen is recommended on the day of the MSLT as the test's validity is affected by the use of recreational drugs.

> **Sleep Latency:** decreased by AntiHistaminics/sedatives/hypnoptics, increased by stimulants
> **Suppressants of REM latency:** Tricyclic antidepressants (TCA's), MAO inhibitors, Amphetamines.
> Hence withdraw these meds 2 weeks before MSLT
> Urine toxicology on am of MSLT. No caffeine, cigarettes, nor ETOH on night before.
> **Indications for MSLT:**
> 1. Narcolepsy
> 2. OSA
> 3. Hypersomnias
> 4. Drug use and need to clear for work
> 5. Insomnia
> 6. Circadian Sleep Disorders
> 7. Assessment of response to therapy. MWT (Maintenance of Wakefulness Test) better.

MAINTENANCE OF WAKEFULNESS TEST (MWT)

The MWT is a variant of MSLT were the patient is asked to stay awake for as long as possible while in the reclining position over 20 to 40 minutes trials. At the first epoch of any stage of sleep the trial is terminated. This test is a better reflection of the ability of a

*ICD-9 codes from the International Classification of Sleep Disorders in parenthesis.

patient to stay awake in a sleep conductive situation and therefore may be a better measure of the patient's alertness in real life situations.

MOOD DISORDERS AND PSG FINDINGS

PSG: Decreased REM latency (normal 70-100' in young adults)
Decreased SWS%

Increased # arousals and ↑ Stage I%=more fragmented sleep.

Increased frequency of eye movements.

Flattening of REM periods length: the length of each REM period increases progressively through the night, making the last one the longest period in normal subjects, but in mood disorders, all the periods tend to be of the same length.

More than 3 REM periods per night suggests narcolepsy.

Average findings in depressed patients: TST is between 5-6 hours, the sleep latency is 30-45', the number of arousals and stage 1% is increased, REM latency and sleep efficiency are decreased, REM periods are flat and there is increased REM density.

Decreased REM density: Dementia, Psychotic depressed (also ↓ REM %).

Endogenous depression: REM latency less than 62' has a sensitivity of 66% and specificity of 79%. However the combination of decreased REM latency, increased REM density and Early Morning Awakening (EMA) has a sensitivity of 77% and specificity of 98%.

Treatment with antidepressants increases sleep time and normalizes to some degree REM periods. During clinical remission without antidepressants, there is no clear increase in the amount and quality of sleep and no normalization of REM sleep.

In primary depression the mean REM latency is 20-40' with more abnormalities than in secondary depression were the mean REM latency is 50-60' with little or no abnormalities in REM.

Antidepressant treatment of major depression half an hour before bedtime:
1. Sedating: Amitriptiline, Trimipramine (no REM effect), Trazodone (suppresses penile detumescence, minimal effect on REM sleep), doxepin.
2. Moderately sedating: Imipramine.
3. Least sedating: desipramine and nortriptiline.
4. Stimulating or non-sedating: Buproprion, Protriptyline and Fluoxetine (Prozac).

ANXIETY DISORDERS

*ICD-9 codes from the International Classification of Sleep Disorders in parenthesis.

- Panic disorder: Somatic symptoms less linked to specific event. Nocturnal panic attacks occur in NREM Stage I, rare at Sleep Onset.
- Obsessive compulsive Disorders
- Phobia
- Generalized anxiety disorder: persistent. Difficulty initiating sleep (DIS), the patient is tired and does not nap.
- Post Traumatic Stress Disorder (PTSD): identifiable trauma, re-experience. DIS if experienced a traumatic event, Difficulty maintaining sleep (DMS) with recollection of trauma and nightmares.

PSG: Increased SO latency, fragmented sleep, decreased SWS.

Differential diagnosis of insomnia secondary to anxiety:
Fifteen percent of patients evaluated at a sleep disorders center have anxiety disorders. The differential diagnosis includes:

1. Psycho physiologic insomnia: anxiety at sleep time only.
2. Major depression: PSG helps to tell the difference. In anxiety disorders we will not find the REM abnormalities found in depression. Both have decreased total sleep time, increase sleep latency and fragmented sleep.
3. Organic causes: nocturnal myoclonus, central sleep apnea, alpha-delta sleep
4. Nocturnal panic attacks must be differentiated from night terrors, nightmares, and sleep chocking syndrome.

Treatment:
1. Behavioral therapy for the phobic and obsessive-compulsive pt.
2. Insight or psychotherapy for general anxiety disorder.
3. If high level of anxiety: benzodiazepines of intermediate duration half an hour before bedtime. Alprazolam, lorazepam and oxazepam, their half-lives are in the range of 8-24 hours. Benzodiazepines of longer action (more than 24 hours), give one dose at bedtime. They include Chlordiazepam, diazepam and Flurazepam. Always start with the smallest dose. May use beta-blockers in anxiety disorders to decrease somatic cardiovascular manifestations. Buspirone is a nonsedating anxiolitic that is a respiratory stimulant during sleep, hence its use in sleep disordered breathing and anxiety.

SCHIZOPHRENIA

1. Abnormal thought processes and hallucinations or delusions.
2. Decreased level of functioning
3. Occurs for longer than 6 months.

PSG:
1. Increased sleep latency.
2. Decreased TST 2-4 hours
3. Decreased REM latency (=mood disorders)
4. Decreased NREM %, especially during the first period. Normal REM %.

*ICD-9 codes from the International Classification of Sleep Disorders in parenthesis.

5. NREM: Decreased%, increased amplitude and amount of delta waves, increased spindles amount and amplitude, increased Stage I, increased number of arousals.
6. There is a decreased tendency for REM rebound after REM sleep deprivation. Phenothiazines improve sleep.

DEMENTIA

PSG:
1. Decreased TST (but not as severe as in depression)
2. Decreased amplitude of delta wave sleep.
3. Fragmented sleep by arousals
4. Decreased REM% but latency is normal or increased, with decreased REM density.
5. K complexes and spindles are decreased in number.

The differential diagnosis includes delirium, affective disorders, drugs, sleep disordered breathing (EDS, awakenings with confusion, wandering, cognitive and personality changes that improve after treatment of OSA).

COMA

PSG findings:
In coma there are delta, alpha, theta and spindles. Nonreactive delta and alpha rhythm carries the worst prognosis. Reactive alpha rhythm carries the best prognosis. If coma persists more than 24 hours, there is worse chance of recovery.

EFFECTS OF MEDICATIONS ON SLEEP AND WAKEFULNESS

HYPNOPTICS
1. **ULTRA RAPID ELIMINATION**
2. Midazolam (Versed), Zolpidem (Ambien) half-life 2-3 hours. Zaleplon (Sonata) peak 1 hour, half life 1 hour.
3. **RAPID ELIMINATION**
   Brotizolam, Zoplicone: Half-life 5 hours.
   The above two groups are hypnotics without residual effects the next day and that do not accumulate on repeated ingestion (except versed).
4. **RELATIVE RAPID ELIMINATION**
   Temazepam (Restoril) soft gel caps peak in 1 hour, half-life 8 hours, hard gel cap peaks in 2 hours, and half-life in 12 hours.
5. **SLOW ELIMINATION**
   Diazepam (Valium) 32 hours, Flunitrazepam (Rohypnol) 15 hours, Flurazepam (Dalmane) 40-103 hours Clorazepate (Tranxene) 63 hours,
6. **SLOW ABSORTION**

*ICD-9 codes from the International Classification of Sleep Disorders in parenthesis.

Lorazepam (Ativan) 8 hours.

ANTIDEPRESANTS (AD)

Sedating AD: They impair performance and produce daytime drowsiness: Amitriptiline, Doxepin, and Mianserin.

Less side effects: Nortriptiline, Clomipramine, Desipramine, protriptiline

↑Psychomotor and cognitive function: Zimelidine and nomifensine (merital) both have been withdrawn from the market, the first one due to its association with Gillain-Barre Syndrome and Merital due to precipitating a serious blood disorder.

Lithium: Salt. Used to treat mania and prevent depression. Increases SWS, mild decrease in REM, may produce atypical sleep stages and at the beginning of therapy it is sedating. During mania and depression, sleep duration is reduced; REM onset latency is also reduced. In mania SWS does not change. Lithium in therapeutic doses inhibits the duration of REM and increases REM latency, SWS increases, wake and drowsy sleep decreases. TST usually does not change. Some times and early on it may produce daytime drowsiness, fatigue and impaired performance.

Neuroleptics: Sedating, they potentiate the effects of alcohol and antihistaminics. Their mechanism of action is inhibition of central DA receptors. Peripheral and central alpha 1 (α1) receptors inhibition leads to sedation and orthostatic hypotension. Phenothiazines, thioxantines, dibenzodiazepines inhibit histamine receptors. The butirophenones (Haldol, spiroperidol), Benzamidas (supliride, senoxipride) and piperazines (trifluperazine, fluphenazine) produce less drowsiness than alkilating phenothiazines (chlorpromazine and promazine). However schizophrenics develop tolerance to drowsiness, therefore there is an increase in psychomotor function and attention with long-term therapy. The effect of Neuroleptics on sleep is complex. Most increase SWS and decrease wakefulness. Chlorpromazine has a dual effect, at low doses it inhibits alpha 2(α2) receptors and increases REM sleep ant high doses decreases REM due to its effects on α1 post synaptic receptors.

Stimulants: Amphetamines: Increased wake and delays onset and duration of REM.

Anorectics: stimulate central Catecholamines leading to insomnia and decrease appetite.

Anticonvulsivants:

Ethosuximide (Zarontin): Increased S1, decreased SWS and REM duration.

Carbamazepine (Tegretol): Decreased REM and decreases the frequency and duration of wakefulness.

Valproic Acid (Depakote): Increases SWS in children, increases drowsy sleep in adults patients. In healthy subjects increases TST, decreases SWS, decreases sleep stage shifts and decreases wakefulness.

Long Term Dilantin: shortens Sleep Onset Latency. There is less drowsiness with Dilantin and Valproic acid.

Antiemetics:

Dopamine antagonists: Metoclopramide, domperidone, phenothiazines all cause drowsiness.

*ICD-9 codes from the International Classification of Sleep Disorders in parenthesis.

Anticholinergics: Scopolamine: short duration of action, increases REM latency, decreases total REM sleep and # of eye movements, increases S2, and produces REM rebound on withdrawal.

5-HydroxiTriptamine: Ondasentron. Used for vomiting in chemotherapy.

Hypnotics or sedative use: decreases alertness, slurred speech, sleepiness and nystagmus.

Dementia: produces alteration of short-term memory, judgment, language and abstract reasoning. Also nocturnal confusion and insomnia.

Tricyclics: Sedating and non-sedating tricyclic antidepressants decrease REM sleep % and increase REM sleep latency.

Sedating: Amitriptiline, doxepin. Administer at HS.

Variable: Imipramine, Nortriptiline.

Exciting: Protriptyline

Reduce or eliminate REM: Clomipramine (Anafranil).

No changes in REM: Trimipramine and Buproprion (increase), Nefazodone (may increase), trazodone (variable), Mirtazapine (variable).

Increase slight in REM: Nefazodone (Serzone).

MAO inhibitors (Phenelzine and Tranylcypromine): overall increase in light sleep at the expense of REM suppression. They are the most powerful REM suppressants. They can't be used with SSRI's or TCA's. REM rebound after abrupt stop of treatment.

Heterocyclic AD –Second Generation:

Inhibitors of the presynaptic reuptake of amines Neurotransmitters:

1) Trazodone (Desyrel): Priapism, very sedating, short elimination rate. Increases SWS, weak reduction in REM. Use with other more activating such as MAO inhibitors and Fluoxetine (Prozac).

Selective serotonin reuptake inhibitors (SSRI's or Serotonin Boosters)
SSRI's have fewer side effects than Tricyclic antidepressants and MAO inhibitors perhaps due to their action on a single neurotransmitter. Sexual side effects are common. Serious side effects (psychosis) if withdrawn abruptly. They decrease REM sleep and increase REM latency. They may increase PLM's /RLS and can induce the REM behavior disorder.

1) Fluoxetine (Prozac): Inhibits Serotonin reuptake. Long duration of action. Alerting, inhibits sleep continuity, anorectic, therefore give it to hypersomniac depressed. At high doses it inhibits REM. Side effects include agitation, anxiety, insomnia, nausea.
2) Paroxetine (Paxil):
3) Sertraline (Zoloft):

*ICD-9 codes from the International Classification of Sleep Disorders in parenthesis.

Mirtazapine (Remeron): 5HT2 blocker (sedation and increased SWS), 5HT3 blocker, Histamine blocker (sedation). Weight gain is a side effect. As hypnotic in low doses (7.5mg to 15 mg at HS). Higher doses 30-45 mg less sedating. Has slight effect in increasing REM sleep. Prolongs REM latency and increases SWS.

Barbiturics: no pain perception if unconscious, no effect if awake. Shorter Sleep Latency, Increased TST, Increase duration and number of Sleep Spindles, decreased REM sleep. REM rebound upon withdrawal of therapy. Barbiturics stimulate hepatic enzymes; hence they decrease the levels of other drugs.

    Long Acting: Phenobarbital, duration of action over 24 hours.

    Intermediate: Amo-, Seco- and Pento-barbital, duration of action 24 hours.

    Short duration: Thiopental, few hours.

Benzodiazepines: Great reduction in SWS, mild reduction in REM, less respiratory depression than barbiturates. They do not induce hepatic enzymes. They decrease sleep latency, increase total sleep time (medium and long acting), decrease to no change in SWS and minor decrease in REM sleep. They also decrease the amplitude of slow waves, increase sigma activity (spindles) and increased high frequency EEG.

Selective Benzodiazepine Receptor Agonists (BZRA): Zolpidem and Sonata. They decrease sleep latency, increase TST, no change to increase in SWS and no change in REM sleep. The effects on EEG activity are similar to the benzodiazepines but less effect on amplitude of slow waves. There is no change in the severity of OSA with Zolpidem and Zaleplon use. (Sleep 200;23 suppl 1, S31-S35). Triazolam (short acting benzodiazepine) on the other hand, decreases the SaO2 sat nadir, but not the mean SpO2 % nor the AHI in severe OSA patients.(Am J Resp Crit Care Med 1995;151:450-454).

Marijuana: initially it causes increased SWS and decreased REM. When used in a chronic basis tolerance develops. Upon withdrawal it increases wake time and increases REM sleep time.

Morphine: Decreased REM sleep.

Hyperthyroidism: Increased SWS.

ANTIPSYCHOTICS GROUPS BY SIDE EFFECTS
1. EXTRAPYRAMIDAL
   Haldol, fluphenazine, trifluoperazine. Use in elderly and HTN.
2. Decreased Blood Pressure, anticholinergics side effects and /or marked sedation. Use in young and agitated patients. Chlorpromazine: Increased SWS (due to -5HT?), decreased Rebound failure of REM, decreased hallucination-like orienting response. Thioridazine.
3. Mixture of 1 and 2. Thiothixene, perphenazine.
4. A mood disorder or personality disorder may not be diagnosed by the referring doctor. Rule out in insomnia with or without sleepiness.
5. Amphetamines, Ritalin (methylphenidate) Pemoline (Cylert) =increase Sleep latency, REM latency, lower TST and REM%.
6. OPIOIDS: decrease TST, S. efficiency and delta & REM sleep.

*ICD-9 codes from the International Classification of Sleep Disorders in parenthesis.

7. Benzodiazepines increase spindle density

INDICATIONS FOR CARDIOPULMONARY SLEEP TESTING (POLYSOMNOGRAPHY)

1. **COPD**: If awake PO2 is greater than 55 mmHg and have evidence of pulmonary hypertension, right heart failure or Polycythemia.
2. **Restrictive Ventilatory Defect:** If illness is complicated by chronic hypoventilation, Polycythemia, pulmonary hypertension, disturbed sleep, morning headache or daytime somnolence and fatigue.
3. **Disorders of respiratory control:** If awake PaCO2 is greater than 45 mmHg or there is evidence of pulmonary hypertension, Polycythemia, disturbed sleep, morning headaches or daytime somnolence and fatigue.
4. **Snoring and or morbid obesity:** with daytime somnolence and or sleep maintenance insomnia and or nocturnal cyclic bradyarrythmias, nocturnal abnormalities of atrioventricular conduction, and ventricular ectopy during sleep that appears increased relative to wakefulness.
5. **Evaluation of sleep complaints:** not explained by history alone.
6. **Evaluation of Erectile Dysfunction:** in the patient with risk factors for OSA, a PSG may be done without an NPT and a therapeutic trial of OSA if present could be performed. Otherwise Nocturnal Penile Tumescence Study could be performed to find out the cause of ED, since there are distinctive features of vascular vs. Neurologic, vs. structural vs. psychogenic causes of ED on NPT study.

TABLES

Table 1. DIFICULTY INITIATING SLEEP DIFFERENTIAL DIAGNOSIS

I.DISOMNIAS

A. Extrinsic
Inadequate Sleep Hygiene (307.41-1)
Environmental sleep disorder (780.52-6)
Sleep- onset association disorder (307.49-4)
Limit-setting sleep disorder   (307.42-4)
Alcohol-dependent sleep disorder (780.52-3)
Toxin-induced sleep disorder (780.54-6)
Extrinsic sleep disorder NOS
Hypnotic-dependent sleep disorder (780.52-8)
Stimulant-dependent sleep disorder   (780.52-1
Food allergy insomnia   (780.52-2)
Adjustment sleep disorder   (307.41-0
Insufficient sleep syndrome   (307.49-4)
 Idiopathic insomnia (780.52-7)

B. Intrinsic
        Psycho physiologic insomnia(307.42-0)
        Sleep state misperception (307.49-1)
        Restless legs syndrome (RLS) (780.52-5)
        Periodic Limb movement disorder (PLMD) (780.52-4)

C. Circadian rhythm sleep disorders
        Time zone change (jet lag) syndrome (307.45-0)

*ICD-9 codes from the International Classification of Sleep Disorders in parenthesis.

Shift work sleep disorder (307.45-1)
Irregular sleep-wake pattern (307.45-3)

II. SLEEP DISORDERS ASSOCIATED WITH
MEDICAL/PSYCHIATRIC
DISORDERS
A. Seep Disorders associated with mental disorders
Anxiety Disorders
Schizophrenia
Mood disorders
B. Sleep disorders associated with neurological disorders
Dementia (331)
Fatal familial insomnia (337.9)

III. PROPOSED SLEEP DISORDERS
Sleep-related neurogenic tachypnea   (780.53-2)
Menstrual Associated sleep disorder (780.54-3)
Pregnancy-associated sleep disorder (780.59-6)

TABLE 2.

MEDICATIONS THAT COMMONLY CAUSE INSOMNIA

1. ß-Blockers
2. Corticosteroids
3. Bronchodilators
4. Respiratory stimulants (theophylline)
5. Stimulating antidepressants
    Protriptyline, fluoxetine, buproprion
6. Methyldopa
7. Thyroid supplements
8. CNS stimulants
9. Decongestants
10. Phenytoin

*ICD-9 codes from the International Classification of Sleep Disorders in parenthesis.

SLEEP DIARY
Patient name:

Date:

Instructions:
Leave blank the periods you are awake.
Mark your bedtime with an arrow pointing downward (↓).
Mark the time you get up in the morning or after naps with arrows pointing upwards (↑).
Fill in the times you are asleep with shaded boxes.
Please note sample in first row, M indicates Monday, this patient went to bed at 10 PM,
was awake twice during the nigh for about one hour at 2 AM and 3 AM,
got up at 6 AM and took an uninterrupted nap for 2 hours from 2 PM to 4 PM.
Enter the initial of the day you started this log and proceed to fill in as in the sample.

Date	1/4													
Hour/Day	M													
MN	▓													
AM	▓													
2														
	▓													
4	▓													
6	↑													
8														
10														
Noon														
PM														
2	↓													
	▓													
4	↑													
6														
8														
10	↓													
	▓													

*ICD-9 codes from the International Classification of Sleep Disorders in parenthesis.

Sample Sleep Study Order Form. Insurance Companies require an indication to perfom sleep studies, so most laboratories have an order form where you can select what condition you suspect and why. This form is used at Sleep ePortal Sleep Disorders Center in Independence, Ohio.

Patient Name_____

Address_____

City_____ State _____ ZIP_____

Home Phone_____ Work Phone_____ E-mail_____

Birthdate_____ Gender ____M____F

Indication
› **Possible OSA**: (please check all that apply)
› Snoring
› Waking up at night choking
› Falling asleep while driving
› Neck circumference more than 17 inches in males and 16 inches in females.
› Hypertension
› Diabetes Mellitus
› BMI more than 29
› Impotence
› Excessive Daytime Sleepiness (EDS)
› History of Obstructive Sleep Apnea (OSA)
› History of OSA treated surgically (UPPP)
› Weight Gain
› Weight Loss
› Pre-Bariatric Surgery
› Post-Bariatric Surgery

› Difficulty initiating sleep
› Difficulty maintaining sleep
› Non-refreshing sleep
› **Possible Narcolepsy**:
› Excessive Daytime sleepiness
› Cataplexy
› Hypnagogic hallucinations
› Sleep paralysis
› Other:
› _____
› _____

COMMENTS / SPECIAL NEEDS
_____
_____
_____
_____

TEST REQUESTED
› Polysomnography (Sleep Study)
› Split night study
› CPAP Titration
› Overnight EEG
› Baseline PSG and MSLT
› Other _____
Priority:
□ **Urgent**
□ **Normal**

INTERPRETING / READING PHYSICIAN
› Dr. Berta Briones
› Dr. Don Wolfson
› Other_____
_____
Clinical management desired
□ Yes
□ No

_____/_____ / _____
Physician Signature /Print name   Date

*ICD-9 codes from the International Classification of Sleep Disorders in parenthesis.

AKNOWLEDGEMENTS

With special thanks to my parents for inspiring me and providing my education, to my mentor, Dr. Sopko for his support in this project and his editorial review, to Dr. Kingman Strohl for his editorial review and to Sister Patricia Marie Thomas, Ingrid and Liesel Sacko for formatting the text and language editing.

Liam Alexander Briones MD, MBA, FAASM, FCCP
November 30th, 2016

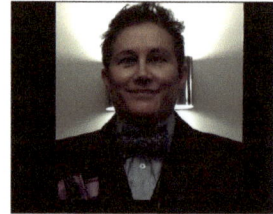

*ICD-9 codes from the International Classification of Sleep Disorders in parenthesis.

www.ingramcontent.com/pod-product-compliance
Lightning Source LLC
Chambersburg PA
CBHW040845180526
45159CB00001B/321